I AM YOUR GIFT

Published by Spines
ISBN: 979-8-89383-922-7

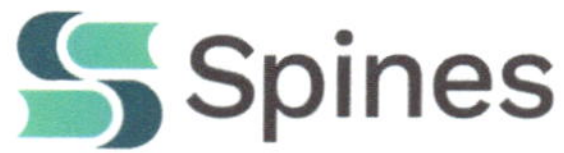

I AM YOUR GIFT

A GUIDE FOR PARENTS AND CAREGIVERS OF SPECIAL NEEDS CHILDREN

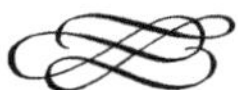

DIANA UWERA

"I gave to the needy when I had nothing, and God blessed me with everything. My heart overflows with joy because there is greater blessing in giving than in receiving. Never fear giving, even when you have little—what you give from the heart will transform your life in ways you can't imagine."

Diana Uwera

ABOUT THE BOOK

Written by Diana Uwera, "I Am Your Gift" is a heartfelt and powerful book dedicated to raising awareness for children with special needs. This book not only provides invaluable insights and practical tips for parents and caregivers but also serves as a voice for the millions of special needs children in Africa who are often overlooked and underserved.

Support a Greater Cause

By purchasing "I Am Your Gift", you are directly contributing to a brighter future for vulnerable children with special needs. The proceeds from this book will help expand support programs, provide essential resources, and ensure that these children receive the care and attention they deserve.

ABOUT THE AUTHOR

Child Protection Advocate.
Human Rights Expert.
Parents, Guardians, Caregivers and Providers of
Children with Special Needs.

TIPS AND GUIDELINES.
2024
ARIZONA-USA

My name is Diana Uwera, and I am a mother and the founder of the International Community Center, dedicated to supporting children with special needs. With over a decade of experience, I have seen the effort, patience, and love this journey requires.

This book, "I Am Your Gift," is my way of helping parents, guardians, caregivers, and providers navigate the unique challenges and rewards of raising a child with special needs. Inside, you'll find tips and insights to guide you through tough times, reminding you to keep going.

Though your child may not always understand the stress or challenges you face, they are a gift—a reminder of the strength you possess. I hope this book offers inspiration and support, empowering you to embrace this journey with courage and love.

A SPECIAL MESSAGE FROM THE AUTHOR

To all the wonderful mothers who dedicate their lives to caring for their special needs children—you are the unsung heroes. I see you. I see the sacrifices you make every day, whether it's missing out on getting your nails done, hanging out with friends, or taking a much-needed vacation. Your love, strength, and dedication are what make the world a better place for your children. You deserve to be recognized, celebrated, and honored by the whole world. Never forget how truly extraordinary you are.

With deep admiration and gratitude,

Diana

A MESSAGE TO PROVIDERS, CAREGIVERS, AND GUARDIANS

Taking care of someone with special needs is a profound and rewarding responsibility, but it can also be incredibly demanding. That's why it's essential to prioritize your mental health and well-being first. Remember, you can't give what you don't have. If you're not filled with passion, love, and kindness, it will be difficult to provide the care and support that your loved ones need and deserve.

This work is not for everyone. It requires immense patience, unwavering love, and a genuine passion for caring. If you find that these qualities do not resonate with you, it's important to consider whether this is the right path. There are many other fields where your talents and skills can make a difference. But for those who are truly called to this work, taking care of yourself is the first and most important step in being able to care for others.

Self-Care and Positivity: Essential Tips for Parents, Providers, Caregivers, and Guardians

To be the best support for your child, it's crucial to take care of yourself too. Here are some key pieces of advice:

- Exercise if You Can: Physical activity can help relieve stress, boost your mood, and improve your overall health. Even a short daily walk can make a big difference.

- Join Support Groups: Connecting with others who understand your journey can provide emotional support, practical advice, and a sense of community. You're not alone in this.

- Stay Positive: Surround yourself with positive influences and avoid negative energy. Your mindset can have a significant impact on your well-being and your child's development.

- Focus on Your Child's Needs: Stay centered on what's most important—your child's growth, happiness, and well-being. By keeping this focus, you can better navigate the challenges and joys of caring for a special needs child.

Here are some uplifting quotes designed to help the parents, caregivers, providers and guardians of special needs children to stay positive through the difficult times.

1. "Your child is not a diagnosis; they are a unique soul with limitless potential."

2. "Embrace the journey, even when it's tough. Your love is the greatest gift you can give."

3. "Focus on the small victories—they are the stepping stones to greater achievements."

4. "Remember, progress is progress, no matter how small. Celebrate every step forward."

5. "Your strength and resilience are an inspiration, even on the days when you feel weakest."

6. "In the midst of challenges, find the beauty in your child's unique way of seeing the world."

7. "You are not alone. There's a community of love, support, and understanding surrounding you."

8. "Sometimes the most difficult roads lead to the most beautiful destinations. Keep going."

9. "You are enough, and so is your child. Together, you can overcome anything."

10. "When it feels like the world is on your shoulders, remember how much your child's smile is worth."

For Those Who Read the Bible

During the most challenging times, remember that God is the greatest and His Word offers comfort and strength. Here are some scriptures that can uplift you:

1. Philippians 4:13: "I can do all things through Christ who strengthens me."

- A reminder that God gives you the strength to overcome any challenge.

2. Isaiah 41:10 : "So do not fear, for I am with you; do not be dismayed, for I am your God. I will strengthen you and help you; I will uphold you with my righteous right hand."

- God promises to be with you and support you, even in the toughest moments.

3. Jeremiah 29:11 : "For I know the plans I have for you," declares the Lord, "plans to prosper you and not to harm you, plans to give you hope and a future."

- Trust in God's plan for you and your child, knowing that He has a purpose filled with hope.

4. Matthew 11:28-30 : "Come to me, all you who are weary and burdened, and I will give you rest. Take my yoke upon you and learn from me, for I am gentle and humble in heart, and you will find rest for your souls. For my yoke is easy and my burden is light."

- When you feel overwhelmed, turn to God for rest and relief.

5. Psalm 46:1 : "God is our refuge and strength, an ever-present help in trouble."

- God is your constant source of strength and protection.

6. Romans 8:28 : "And we know that in all things God works for the good of those who love him, who have been called according to his purpose."

- Even in difficult times, trust that God is working everything for your good.

7. 2 Corinthians 12:9 : "But he said to me, 'My grace is sufficient for you, for my power is made perfect in weakness.' Therefore I will boast all the more gladly about my weaknesses, so that Christ's power may rest on me."

- God's grace is all you need, and His power is strongest when you feel weakest.

A MESSAGE FROM OMAR HABANABAKIZE

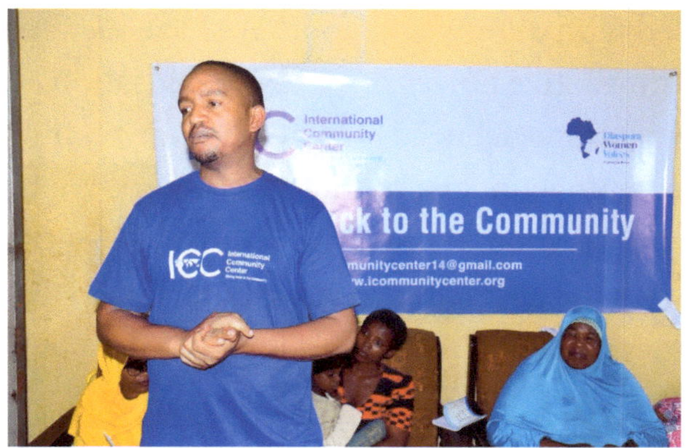

To all readers of this wonderful book "I am your gift " for special needs children in Rwanda and other parts of the World,

As the president of International Community Center in Rwanda, it is my distinct honor to contribute to this important book on children with special needs. Our organization has dedicated itself to advocating for, supporting, and empowering these remarkable children and their families. Through our work, we have witnessed their incredible strength, resilience, and potential.

Children with special needs hold a unique place in our society. They remind us of the diversity of human experience and the beauty of different abilities. It is our collective responsibility to ensure that they receive the support, respect, and opportunities they deserve.

At ICC Rwanda, we believe that every child, regardless of their abilities, has the right to education, healthcare, and a life filled with dignity and hope. We have seen firsthand the transformative power of inclusive education, where children with special needs learn alongside their peers, fostering mutual understanding and respect. We have also seen the profound impact of accessible healthcare and rehabilitation services in improving the quality of life for these children and their families.

This book is a testament to the progress we have made and a reminder of the work that still lies ahead. It is a call to action for all of us—government officials, educators, healthcare professionals, community members, and fellow NGOs—to continue working together to create an inclusive society where every child can thrive.

Let us continue to advocate for policies that promote inclusivity, invest in training and resources for educators and healthcare providers, and raise awareness about the importance of social inclusion. Let us support families, empower individuals with special needs, and celebrate their achievements.

Together, we can build a Rwanda where every child, regardless of their abilities, has the opportunity to reach their full potential. This is our mission, our passion, and our unwavering commitment.

With hope and determination, our organization has been dedicated to improving the lives of these remarkable children, and I am continually inspired by their resilience, strength, and potential.

Children with special needs are an integral part of our community, and it is our collective responsibility to ensure they receive the support, respect, and opportunities they deserve. This book highlights their stories, challenges, and triumphs, serving as both a testament to their spirit and a call to action for all of us.

Rwanda has made significant strides in recent years, but there is still much work to be done. We must continue to advocate for inclusive education, accessible healthcare, and social acceptance. It is through these efforts that we can create a society where every child, regardless of their abilities, can thrive and contribute meaningfully.

I hope this book will inspire you to join us in our mission. Together, we can make a difference in the lives of children with special needs and build a brighter, more inclusive future for all.

Sincerely,

Omar HABANABAKIZE

President, ICC RWANDA

Dear Reader,

Thank you for choosing to purchase *I Am Your Gift*. This book was written from the heart, with a deep passion for supporting and uplifting children with special needs and their families. By opening these pages, you are not only gaining insight into the unique challenges and joys of raising a child with special needs but also joining a community of compassionate individuals who believe in the value and potential of every child.

This book is more than just a collection of words; it is a testament to the strength, resilience, and love that parents of special needs children embody every day. My hope is that you will find guidance, comfort, and inspiration within these pages and that you will feel empowered to advocate for the children in your life and community.

Thank you for your support, and welcome to this journey of understanding, acceptance, and advocacy. Together, we can make a difference in the lives of these incredible children.

With gratitude,

Diana Uwera

CONTENTS

THE JOURNEY OF DIANA AS A HOST HOME PROVIDER

Since 2015, my life has been profoundly transformed by my journey as a host home provider. There's something truly life-changing about witnessing the transformation of someone in your care, knowing that it's your dedication, love, and commitment to providing care with dignity that has made all the difference. The fulfillment that comes from learning new ways to offer quality care and seeing the positive impact it has on another person's life is beyond words.

As a single mother, I chose to open my home to individuals with special needs. This decision allowed me to be a blessing to someone else while also providing the best possible care and guidance to my own children in a world that can often be harsh and unpredictable. The experience has been nothing short of extraordinary.

I encourage anyone with a loving heart to consider stepping into this role. Being a host home provider is an opportunity to change someone's life in ways you can't even imagine. However, it's important to understand that this work requires more than just time and effort—it demands a deep passion for helping others. If you don't truly love and care for humanity, this might not be the path for you. But for those who do, the rewards are immeasurable.

Over the years, the people I've cared for have become a part of my life, my family, and my heart. The bonds we've formed are strong and meaningful, and I am deeply grateful for the opportunity to share my home and my life with them.

If you're looking for a way to make a real difference in the world, to bring comfort and joy to someone who needs it most, I invite you to consider becoming a host home provider. It's a commitment that requires love, patience, and dedication, but the impact you can have on another person's life—and the fulfillment you will feel in your own—makes it all worthwhile.

For parents who have devoted themselves to raising their children with special needs, I want to offer words of encouragement: never give up. However, when it comes to making decisions for your adult son or daughter, you may want to consider options like an Adult Developmental Home or a Child Developmental Home.

These are specialized environments led by trained professionals who have chosen to open their homes to individuals with special needs, ensuring they still feel at home, even when they are away from their families.

It's important to remember that as a parent, you continue to play a vital role in making decisions for your child. Many parents choose these developmental homes to give their children the chance to learn and grow in ways that prepare them for a world beyond the familiarity of home. We live in a world where a special needs child often forms a deep attachment to their mother, but it's equally important that they are given opportunities to learn, explore, and develop independence.

Many parents make this decision to help their children adapt to life without them while still maintaining strong family ties. Children or adults in developmental homes still visit home and participate in family events and holidays, preserving that essential connection.

If you find yourself mentally exhausted, dealing with medical issues, or simply in need of support, please consider the option of developmental homes. There are agencies available to guide you through the entire process. For more information, feel free to email me at <u>dianauwera@yahoo.com</u>.

INTRODUCTION

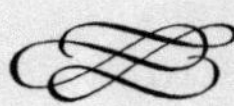

First of all, who is a special needs child? A special needs child is a child/youth who has been determined to require special attention and specific necessities that other children do not.

Special needs can also be a legal designation.

Particularly in the adoption and foster care community, where in the child and guardian receive support to help them both lead productive lives. That applies in USA and some other developed continents like Europe and Australia but in Africa, parents don't have any sort of resource or support for children with special needs and it's very concerning because parents with special needs in African countries have to go through a lot in life, some are humiliated by the society and family members. They are being mocked that they have possessed children and that result them to hide their children so no one should see them.

Most of then end up being single mothers because their husbands run away for fearing what people will say about them having children with special needs. The society call them abnormal children and every abnormal child belongs to the mother in most African cultures.

In my opinion, this has to stop. All women get pregnant for nine month or less depending on every woman's condition not knowing who they will give birth to but if it happens and you receive a child with special needs, know that God selected you among billions of people on this earth to be the mother and father of that child.

Dear mothers, don't feel sorry for anything, just ask God to give you strength to love and care for your child because that child is going to need you forever.

You are the only person she/he is looking up to. You are their only hope, that's why mother's love is unconditional.

God chose you for a reason and he is ready to guide you and to give you strength to raise that child no matter the challenges and circumstances you are going through as a parent.

Raising a child with special needs can involve so many challenges, but, there are many ways to support them and help them become successful, independent and have confidence.

I have shared with you some tips that can help you in raising a child with special needs.

- Get to know your child: Try to understand their personalities, what they like and dislike and what makes them happy or sad.
- Learn about their condition: Knowing their condition can help you identify potential medical issues, support their development, and advocate for them.
- Create a routine: Children with special needs may benefit from structure and routine, which can help reduce anxiety and increase their sense of security.
- Advocate for your child: Speaking up for your child can help them get the support, services and accommodations they need.
- Be inclusive: Educate family, friends, and peers about your child's needs to help foster understanding and acceptance.
- Find support: You can connect with other parents of children with special needs through online communities, blogs, and support groups.

You can also seek support from parents who understand what you are going through.

Don't be isolated, get out, meet other parents, sit and talk, share experiences and some tips on how you can make a difference in your children's lives. Sometimes you need that person who can listen to you, who understands what you are going through, it will release that pain, that stress, knowing that you are not alone.

- Take care of yourself: Make sure you are getting enough sleep, eating healthy foods, exercising regularly, and finding time to relax and de-stress.
- Be patient: Try to focus on the small milestones your child achieves instead of dwelling on the bigger challenges.

AUTISM

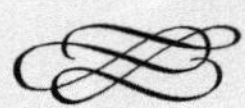

Autism is a developmental special need that significantly affects verbal and non-verbal communication and social interaction, generally evident before age three, that adversely affects a child's educational performance.

Other characteristics often associated with Autism are engaged in repetitive activities and stereotyped movements, resistance to environmental change or change in daily routines, and unusual responses to sensory experience.

The term doesn't apply if a child's educational performance is adversely affected primarily because the child has an emotional disturbance as defined in this section.

The term of Autism also includes students who have been diagnosed with an autism spectrum disorder such as Autism- Pervasive Developmental Disorder- Not otherwise specified (PDD-NOS) or a Sperger's syndrome when the child's education performance is adversely affected. Additionally, it may also include diagnosis of a Pervasive Developmental Disorder such as Rett's Childhood Disintegrative Disorder.

Autism may exist concurrently with other areas of special needs.

After age three, a child could be diagnosed as having Autism if the child manifests the above characteristics.

Children with Autism demonstrate the following characteristics prior to age three.

- Difficulty relating to others or interacting in a socially appropriate manner.
- Absence, disorder or delay in verbal and/or non-verbal communication; and
- One or more of the following:

1. Insistence on sameness as evidence by restricted play patterns, repetitive body movements, persistent or unusual preoccupations, and/or resistance to change.
2. Unusual or Inconsistent responses to sensory stimuli.
3. Evaluation: The characteristics identified in the Autism definition are present.

Evaluation procedures

Evaluation of Autism shall include the following;

- Parental interviews including developmental history.
- Behavioral observations in two or more settings
- (can be two settings within the school)
- Physical and neurological information from a licensed physician, pediatrician or neurologist who can provide general health history to evaluate the possibility of other impacting health conditions.

Evaluation participants

Information shall be gathered from the following persons in the evaluation of autism spectrum disorders.

- The parent;
- The child's general education classroom teachers (with a child less than school age, an individual qualified to teach a child of his/her age);
- A licensed special education teacher;
- A licensed school psychologist, licensed psychologist examiner (under the direct supervision of a licensed psychologist), licensed

senior psychological examiner, or licensed psychiatrist;

- A licensed physician, neurologist, paediatrician or primary care provider;
- A certified speech/language teacher or specialist; and
- Other professional personnel as needed, such as an occupational therapist, physical therapist or guidance counsellor.

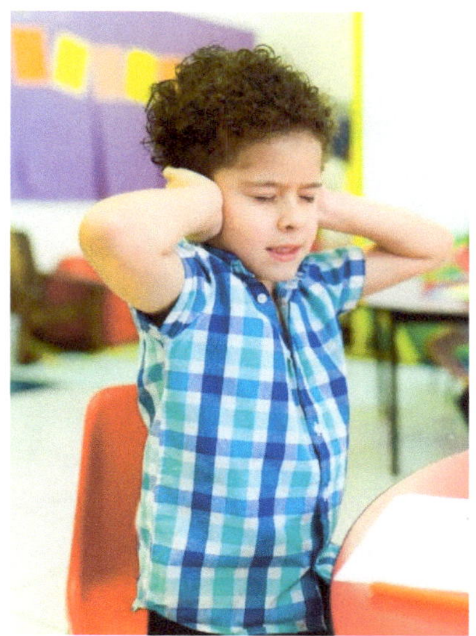

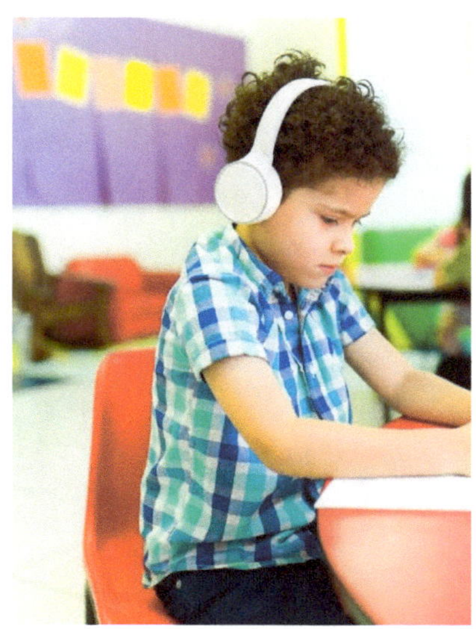

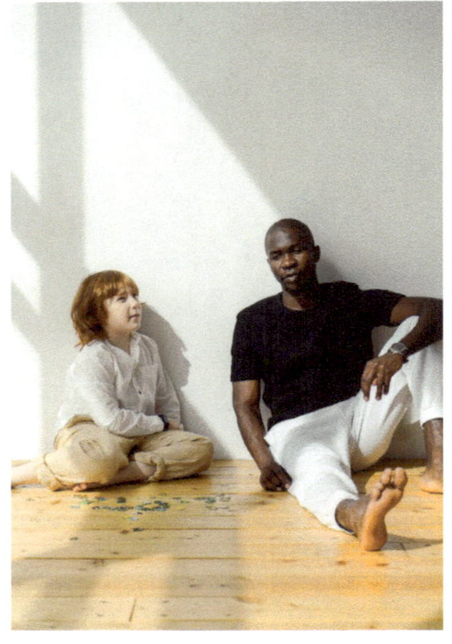

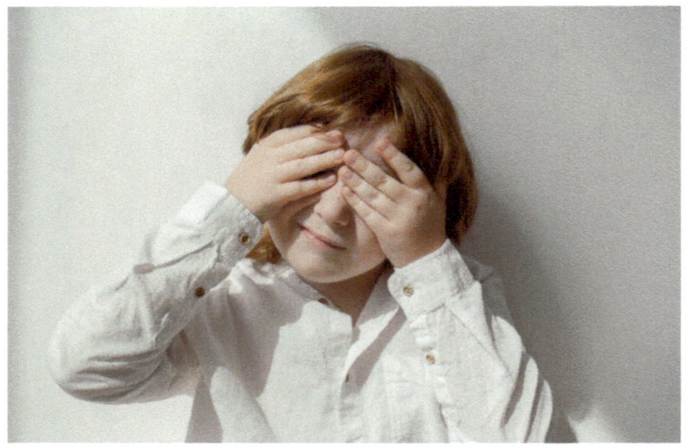

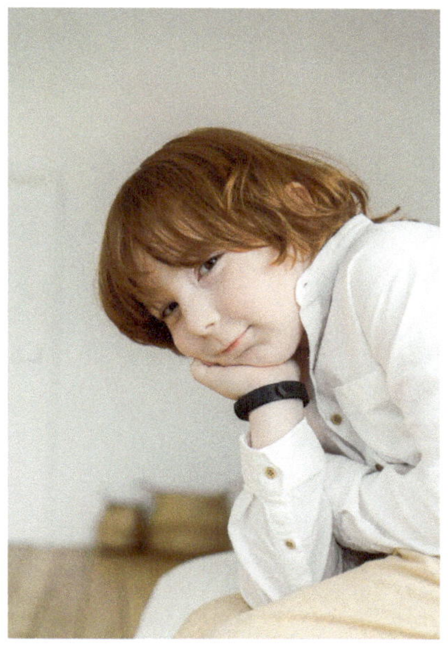

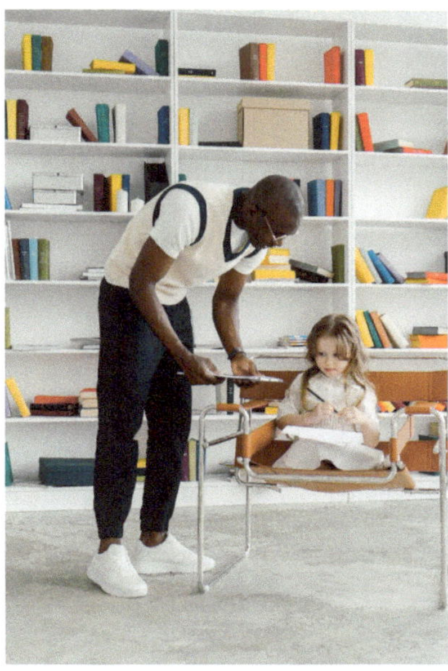

DEAFNESS AND BLINDNESS

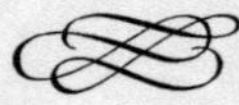

Deafness and blindness mean concomitant hearing and visual impairments, the combination of which, causes such severe communication and other developmental and educational needs that they cannot be accommodated in special education programs by addressing any one of the impairments. A child with deaf-blindness shall have at least one of the following;

- A child who meets criteria for Deafness/Hearing Impairment and Visual Impairment.
- A child who is diagnosed with a degenerative condition or syndrome which lead to Deaf-Blindness, affected by both hearing and vision deficits; or
- A child with severe multiple special needs due to generalized central nervous system dysfunction,

and who exhibits auditory and visual, impairments or deficits which are not perceptual in nature.

Evaluation

The characteristic identified in the Deaf-Blindness definition are present.

Evaluation procedures

Evaluation of Deaf-Blindness shall include the required evaluation procedures for hearing impairments/deafness and visual impairment and include the following;

1. Deafness/Hearing Impairment procedures

- Audiological evaluation.
- Evaluation of speech and language performance.
- School history and levels of learning or educational performance.
- Observation of the child's auditory functioning and classroom performance; and
- Documentation, including observation and or assessment, of how Deafness/Hearing Impairment adversely impacts the child's educational performance in his/her learning environment.

2. Visual Impairment Procedures

- Eye exam and evaluation completed by an Ophthalmologist or Optometrist that documents the eye condition with the best possible correction and includes a description of etiology diagnosis, and prognosis of the visual impairment evaluation.
- A written functional vision and media assessment, completed or compiled by a licensed teacher of students with visual impairments that includes
- Observation of Visual behaviors at school, home or other environments.
- Education implications of eye condition based upon the information received from eye report.
- Assessment and/or screening of expanded core curriculum skills (orientation and mobility, social interaction, visual efficiency, independent living)

Special need Eligibility Standard 4.

Recreation and leisure, career education, assistive technology, and compensatory skills as well as an evaluation of the child's reading and writing skills, needs, appropriate reading and writing media, and current and future needs for Braille (Braille is a technology that allows blind and partially sighted people to learn spelling, grammar and punctuation and gain an understanding of how text is formatted on the page).

- School history and levels of educational performance.

Documentation

Including observation and/or assessment, of how visual impairment adversely affects educational performance in the classroom or learning environment.

- Evaluation of a child with suspected degenerative condition or syndrome which will lead to Deaf-Blindness shall include a medical statement confirming the existence of such a condition or syndrome and its prognosis.

Additional evaluation of Deaf-Blindness shall include the following;

- Expanded core curriculum skills assessment that includes Deafness/Hearing Impairment.
- Assessment of speech and language functioning including the child's mode of communication.
- Documentation, including observation and/or assessment, of how Deaf-Blindness adversely impacts the child's educational performance in his/her learning environment.

Evaluation Participants

Information shall be gathered from the following persons in the evaluation of Deaf-Blindness;

- The parent.
- The child's general education classroom teacher,
- A licensed physician or audiologist.
- A licensed speech/language teacher or specialist.
- An ophthalmologist or optometrist.
- A licensed teacher of students with visual impairments; and
- Other professional personnel, as indicated example (low vision specialist, orientation, and mobility instructor, school psychologist.

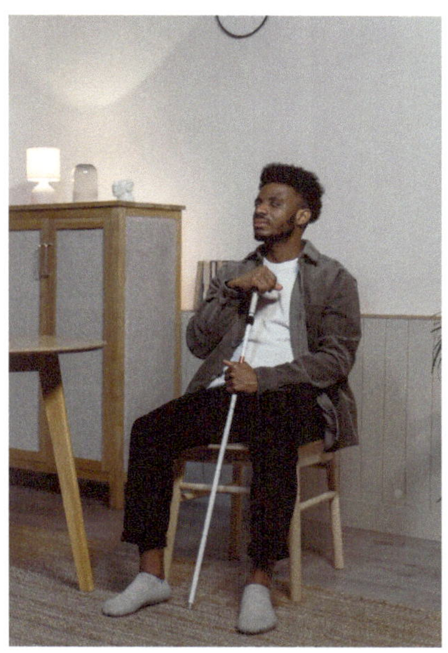

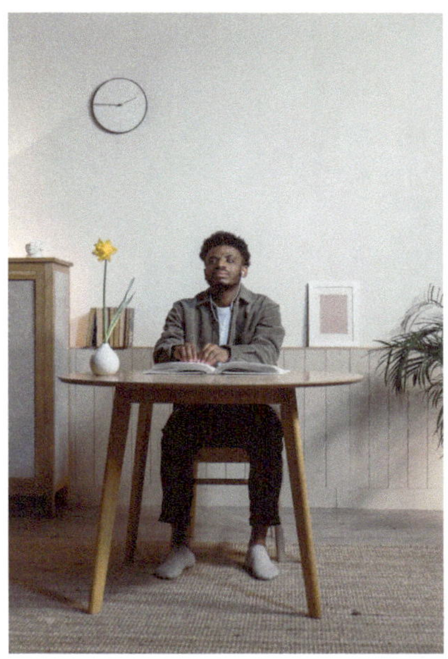

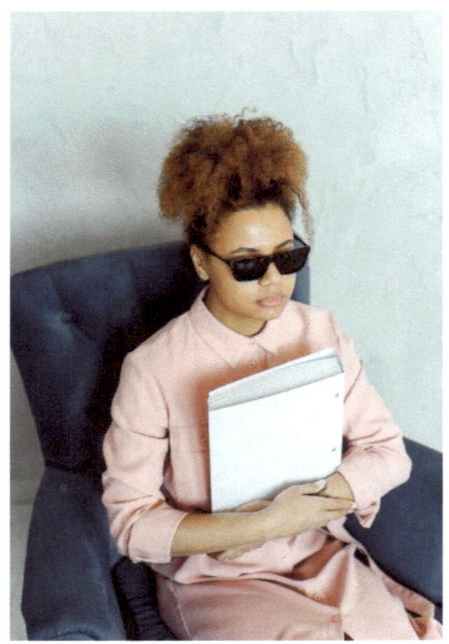

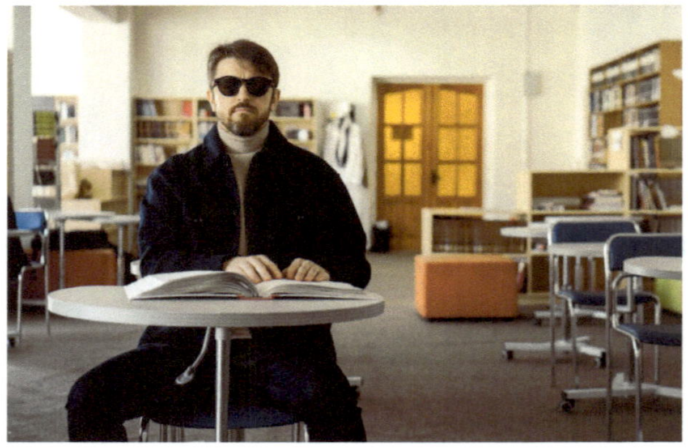

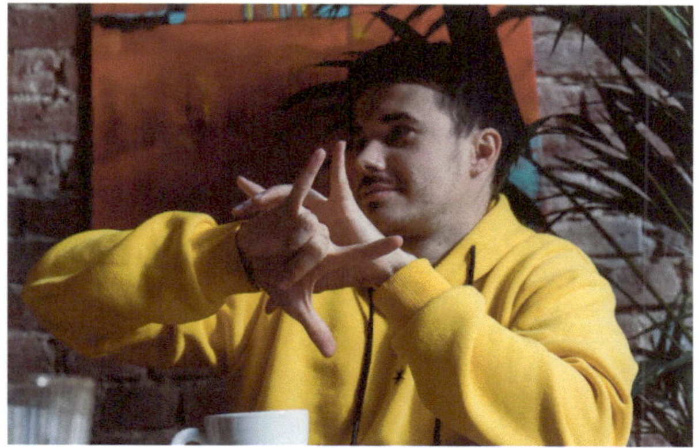

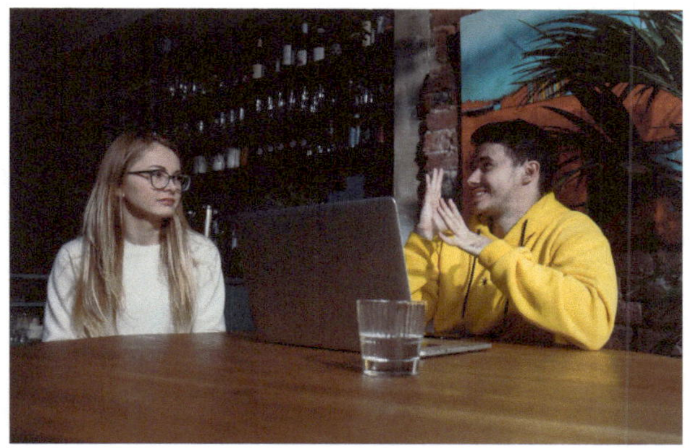

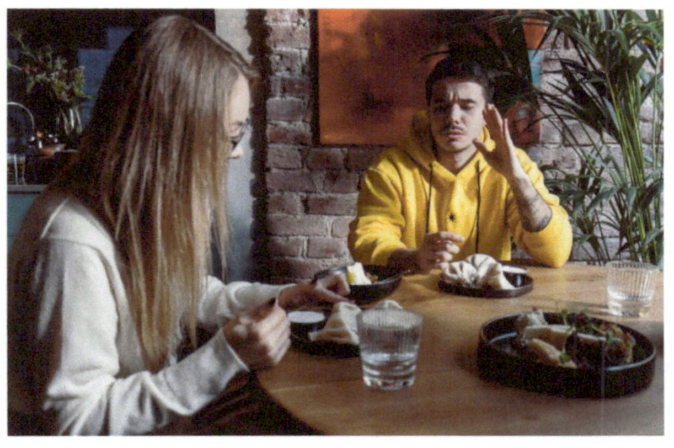

DOWN SYNDROME

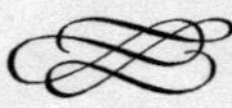

Down syndrome is a genetic chromosome 21 disorder causing developmental and intellectual delays. It is also a genetic disorder caused when abnormal cell division results in extra genetic material from chromosome 21.

Down syndrome causes a distinct facial appearance Intellectual special need, developmental delays and may be associated with thyroid or heart disease.

What does Down Syndrome affect?

Down syndrome can affect anyone. It's a genetic condition, and it doesn't happen as a result of something that the parents did before or during pregnancy.

The majority of Down Syndrome cases happen randomly (sporadically).

People don't usually inherit Down Syndrome in an

autosomal dominant or recessive pattern during conception when the egg and sperm meet.

As parents of special needs child with Down Syndrome, don't blame yourselves, you didn't do anything wrong. It comes naturally.

Symptoms and Causes

Down Syndrome causes physical, cognitive and behavioral symptoms. Not all people with Down Syndrome have all of these symptoms.

Symptoms and their severity are different from person to person.

Physical signs of Down Syndrome

Physical signs of Down syndrome are usually present at birth and become more apparent as your baby grows.

They can include;

- A flat nose bridge.
- Slanted eyes that point upward.
- A short neck.
- Small ears, hand and feet.
- Weak muscle tone at birth.
- Small pinky finger that points inward towards the thumb.
- One crease in the palm of their hand (palmar crease)

- Shorter-than average height.

As your child grows, additional symptoms can arise because of the way that their body developed in the uterus, including;

- Ear infection or healing loss.
- Dental problems.
- Being more prone to infections or illnesses.
- Obstructive sleep apnea.
- Congenital heart disease.

Your child's health care provider will regularly check for these and other conditions that may cause additional symptoms throughout your child's life.

Cognitive Symptoms of Down Syndrome

Your child with Down Syndrome may have cognitive development challenges as a result of their extra chromosome. This can cause Intellectual or special needs.

Your child's ability to meet developmental milestones, or things that your child can do at a certain age, may differ from other children, including how they:

- Walk and move (gross and fine motor skills)
- Speak (language development skills)
- Learn (cognitive skills)

- Play (social and emotional skills)

As a result, it may take your child longer to do the following things:

- Toilet training.
- Speaking their first words.
- Taking their first steps.
- Eating food independently.

Behavioral Symptoms of Down Syndrome

Your child diagnosed with Down Syndrome may exhibit behavioral symptoms. This can be the result of your child not being able to communicate their needs to you or their caregivers effectively.

Behavioral symptoms of Down Syndrome could include;

- Stubbornness and tantrums.
- Difficulty paying attention.
- Obsessive or compulsive behaviors.

Diagnosis and Tests

How is Down Syndrome diagnosed before birth?

A healthcare provider can suspect Down Syndrome during pregnancy with prenatal screening tests. They can also diagnose this condition during pregnancy with diagnostic tests.

Prenatal Screening tests

These tests assess your risk of having a child with down syndrome rather than giving you a confirmation of diagnosis. Screening tests could be a blood test of the birthing parent's blood to look for indicators of Down Syndrome.

Another screening test is an ultra sound. During this imaging test, your provider will look for signs of Down Syndrome like extra fluid behind your baby's neck.

It's possible that a screening test could be normal and not show signs of Down Syndrome when the condition is present.

What if I find out that the foetus has Down Syndrome?

If you find out the foetus you are carrying has Down Syndrome, your provider will direct you to resources to help you after the birth of your baby. You may want to participate in counselling or join a support group.

Counsellors and support groups help you prepare for raising a child with Down Syndrome.

In support groups, you can talk with other parents about their experiences raising a child with Down Syndrome.

It's a great way to share practical advice on managing the condition, it's frustration and joys.

These groups offer a sense of belongings and give you support, so you know you are not alone.

In Africa they don't have enough resources, children with special needs are helpless that's why me and my team are working so hard to advocate for children with special needs so our voices can be heard and get them support and enough resources so parents can be able to take good care of their children.

After carefully reviewed how parents go through a lot even in developed countries like United States of America where children with special needs have rights to attend schools, attend Olympic games, have good healthcare access, food (special diet) speech and occupational therapists, physical therapy, counselling and other resources, I decided to focus on children in Africa.

I started with Rwanda where we have many children in our program and others are on waiting list to get help, support or someone who can sponsor their needs. Our program helps children with special needs to get some basic needs and we also help some mothers to start small businesses while watching their children. Our goal is to open a big centre where children can spend at least 6 hours a day learning, playing and enjoying the new environment with Special Education team that includes teachers, therapists, sign language teachers and counsellors.

You can support children with special needs in financial wise but parents need emotional support, words of encouragement and someone to talk to and someone who can listen to them and comfort them.

Those parents in Rwanda go through a lot to the point where they decided to hide their children from society especially people who mock them for having children with conditions, but there are good people also who reach out and encourage them not to give up on their children.

The aim of this book is to let parents with special needs children know that they are not alone and to let them know that they are super heroes and wonder women and God loves them.

In this journey of supporting children with special needs, I have witnessed good people who could walk miles away to go visit those families, talk to them and give them hope for tomorrow.

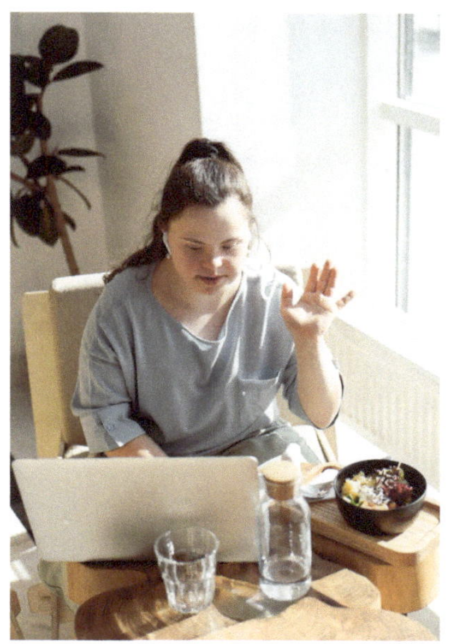

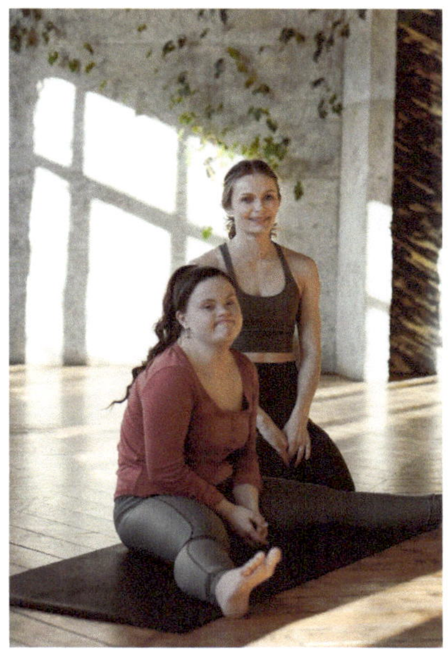

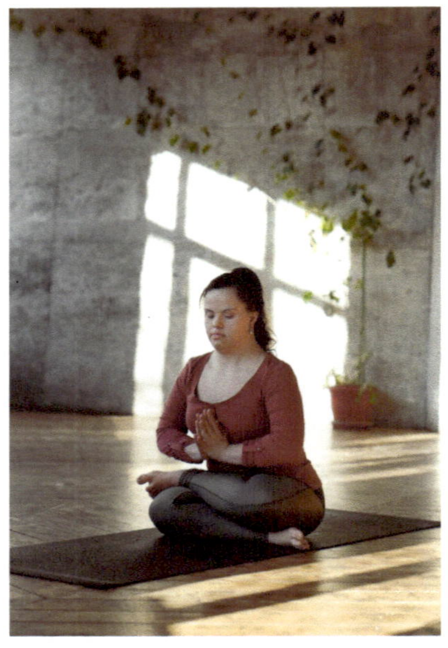

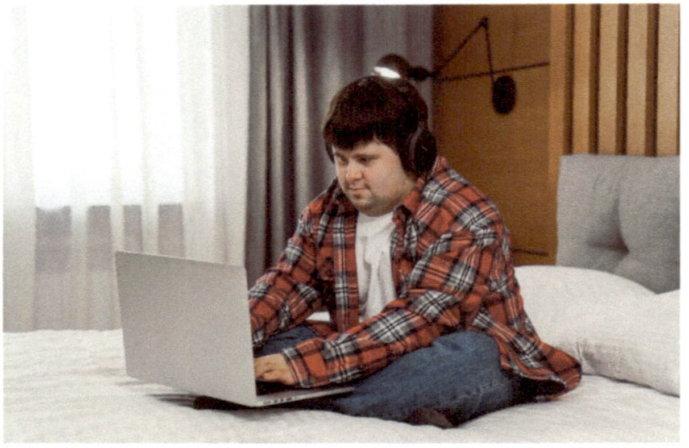

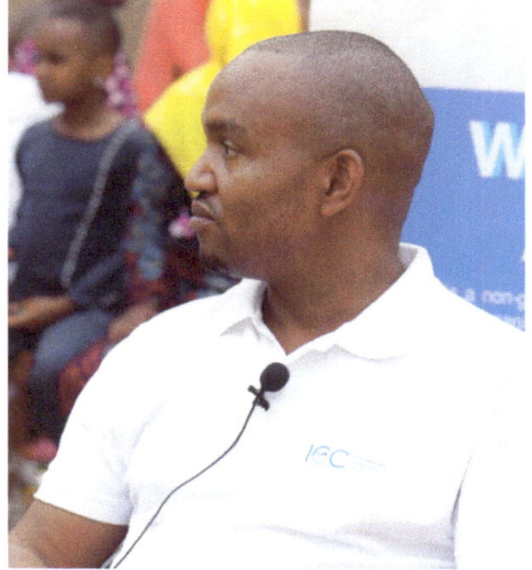

Omar Habanabakize

A special thanks to Omar Habanabakize, the President of International Community Center (ICC) in Rwanda who made an impact in the lives of children with special needs and their parents by reaching out them and making sure their needs are met.

I also want to recognize Laurence Umuhoza, a woman activist, an advocate, and a Nurse Practitioner in the mental health department. She works closely with the mothers of children with special needs and makes sure she communicates with them; they are open to her because she is a good listener.

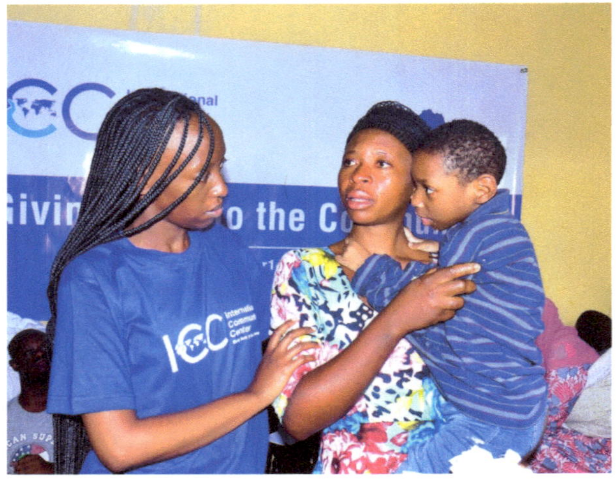

Laurence Umuhoza

Here is a message from Laurence:

"My name is Laurence Umuhoza, and I am a dedicated Gender Advocate, public and mental health practitioner with a special focus on supporting parents of children with special needs. With 5 years of experience in the field working with women, I have had the privilege of working with many families, helping them navigate the unique challenges and joys that come with raising a child with special needs.

I understand that parenting a child with special needs can be both immensely rewarding and incredibly demanding. My goal is to provide a compassionate and supportive environment where they can explore their feelings, gain valuable coping strategies, and find the strength to advocate for their child effectively.

My approach is holistic, integrating evidence-based practices with a deep respect for their personal experiences and insights. I offer individual counseling, support groups, and workshops designed to address the specific emotional and psychological needs of parents.

Whether they need someone to talk to, practical advice, or a supportive community, I am here to help. Together, we can work towards enhancing their well-being and ensuring that their child thrives.

My supportive message

Dear Parents,

I want to take a moment to acknowledge the incredible journey you are on with your child. Parenting is a challenging and rewarding experience for everyone, but raising a child with special needs brings unique joys and challenges that only a select few can truly understand.

Your dedication, love, and resilience are truly remarkable. Every day, you face and overcome obstacles that many cannot even imagine, and you do so with grace and unwavering strength. Your child is lucky to have you as their advocate and protector, ensuring they have the support and opportunities they need to thrive.

It's important to remember that you are not alone. There is a community of parents, professionals, and organizations ready to support you and your child. Seek out those connections, share your experiences, and lean on others when you need to.

Your well-being is just as important as your child's, and taking care of yourself ensures you can be the best possible support for them.

Celebrate every milestone, no matter how small it may seem. Your child's progress is a testament to their incredible spirit and your unwavering support. Each step forward is a victory worth celebrating.

Please know that your efforts do not go unnoticed. Your love and dedication make a profound difference in your child's life, and you are doing an amazing job. Continue to believe in yourself and your child, and know that you are making a positive impact every single day.

With heartfelt admiration and support,

As a Mental health practitioner

Dear Parents,

My name is Laurence Umuhoza, and I am a mental health practitioner dedicated to supporting families like yours. I understand that raising a child with special needs brings unique challenges and extraordinary rewards. Your journey, filled with both triumphs and trials, is one that requires immense strength, patience, and love.

I am here to provide the emotional support and practical guidance you need to navigate this path. My role is to be a compassionate ally, helping you manage stress, find balance, and celebrate the milestones along the way. Together, we can explore strategies to enhance your well-being and empower you to be the best advocate for your child.

Parenting a child with special needs often means facing complex emotions and situations. You might feel overwhelmed, isolated, or uncertain about the future. Please know that you are not alone. My services include individual counseling, support groups, and workshops tailored to address the specific needs of parents like you.

Your dedication to your child's growth and happiness is inspiring. Every small step forward is a victory, and every challenge overcome is a testament to your resilience and love. I am here to support you in every way I can, providing a safe space to share your experiences, seek advice, and find comfort.

Thank you for allowing me to be a part of your journey. Together, we can work towards creating a positive and nurturing environment for you and your child.

We have Umuganwa Asiimwe Diane who is always available to give a hand to help children with special needs and their parents in Rwanda."

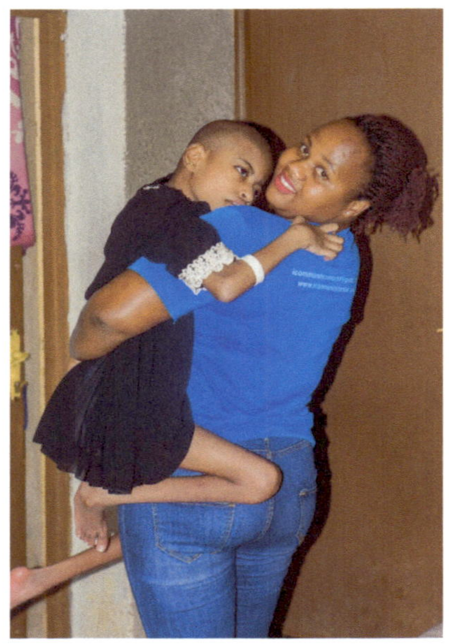

Diane Asiimwe Umuganwa

Here is Diane's message as well:

"I am umuganwa Asiimwe Diana secretary officer at ICC Rwanda, we experienced and motivated special needs education professional with a history of innovation and driving successful program for special needs seeking challenging carriers advancing special needs child emotional, physical and mental needs, parenting a child with special needs can be challenging, but it can also be gratifying. These children require extra care and attention, but with the right mindset and approach, parents can create a fulfilling life for their children and themselves. through Educating yourself: about your special needs child is essential to provide the best possible care and support.

Patient:

Being patient with a special needs child can be challenging but crucial to their development and well-being. First, it's essential to understand their individual needs, abilities, and limitations.

Embrace Your Child's Differences: Embracing your special needs child's differences is essential to creating a positive and inclusive environment that supports their growth and well-being. First, focus on your child's <u>strengths and abilities</u> rather than their limitations.

Advocate for Your Child: *As a parent, it's your job to advocate for your child.*

Emphasize Play and Socialization: *Play and socialization are crucial for all children, including those with special needs. Please encourage your child to engage in play and social activities to help them develop essential social skills and build relationships.*

In conclusion, parenting a special needs child requires patience, understanding, and support. By educating yourself, creating a support network, setting realistic goals, and emphasizing play and socialization, you can help your child succeed. Additionally, ICC can be an excellent resource for improving your child's coordination and motor skills while providing parents with support and guidance. Remember that parenting a special needs child is a journey; with the right mindset and approach, it can be incredibly fulfilling.

In USA, I want to thank two wonderful women who went beyond to make sure the lives of children with special needs in Rwanda are transformed and changed for better and these mothers of special needs children in Rwanda are forever grateful to have such wonderful people like you who thought of them and make their dream lives come to reality.

Nadia, thank you for visiting these women in Rwanda and thanks for everything you do to make their lives easy.

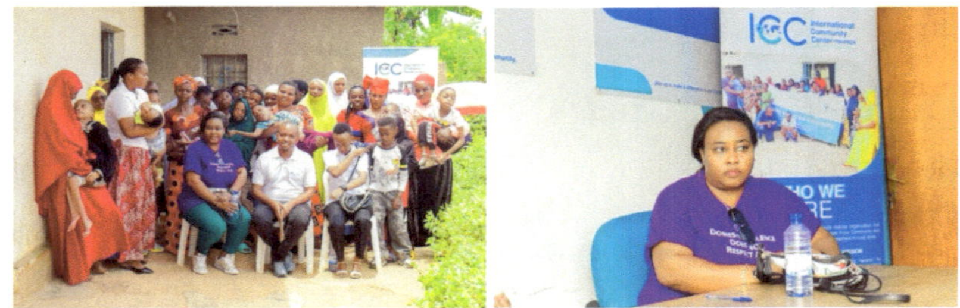

Nadia

Trinh, thank you for everything you have done for these mothers by sponsoring them to start small businesses to be able to provide for their children.

May God bless you.

We need more people like Trinh to change the lives of vulnerable people in the World."

CEREBRAL PALSY

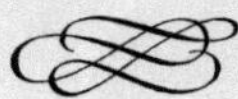

Cerebral palsy is a group of conditions that affect movement and posture. It's caused by damage that occurs to the developing brain, most often before birth.

Symptoms appear during infancy or preschool years and vary from very mild to serious. Children with cerebral palsy may have exaggerated reflexes. The arms, legs and trunk may appear floppy. Or they may have stiff muscles, known as spasticity. Symptoms also can include irregular posture, movements that can't be controlled, a walk that's not steady or some combination of these.

Advertisement

Cerebral palsy may make it hard to swallow. It also can cause eye muscle imbalance, in which the eyes don't focus on the same object. People with the condition might have reduced range of motion in their joints due to muscle stiffness.

The cause of cerebral palsy and its effect on function vary from person to person. Some people with cerebral palsy can walk while others need assistance. Some people have intellectual disabilities, but others do not. Epilepsy, blindness or deafness also might affect some people with cerebral palsy. There is no cure, but treatments can help improve function. The symptoms of cerebral palsy may vary during the child's development, but the condition doesn't get worse. The condition generally stays the same over time.

Symptoms

Symptoms of cerebral palsy can vary greatly. In some people, cerebral palsy affects the whole body. In other people, symptoms might only affect one or two limbs or one side of the body. General symptoms include trouble with movement and coordination, speech and eating, development, and other issues.

Movement and coordination

Movement and coordination symptoms may include:

• Stiff muscles and exaggerated reflexes, known as spasticity. This is the most common movement condition related to cerebral palsy.

• Variations in muscle tone, such as being either too stiff or too floppy.

• Stiff muscles with regular reflexes, known as rigidity.

• Lack of balance and muscle coordination, known as ataxia.

• Jerky movements that can't be controlled, known as tremors.

• Slow, writhing movements.

• Favoring one side of the body, such as only reaching with one hand or dragging a leg while crawling.

• Trouble walking. People with cerebral palsy may walk on their toes or crouch down when they walk. They also may have a scissors-like walk with their knees crossing. Or they may have a wide gait or a walk that's not steady.

• Trouble with fine motor skills, such as buttoning clothes or picking up utensils.

Speech and eating

These symptoms related to speech and eating may occur:

• Delays in speech development.

• Trouble speaking.

• Trouble with sucking, chewing or eating.

• Drooling or trouble with swallowing.

Development

Some children with cerebral palsy have these symptoms related to development:

• Delays in reaching motor skills milestones, such as sitting up or crawling.

• Learning disabilities.

• Intellectual disabilities.

• Delayed growth, resulting in smaller size than would be expected.

Other symptoms

Damage to the brain can contribute to other neurological symptoms, such as:

• Seizures, which are symptoms of epilepsy. Children with cerebral palsy may be diagnosed with epilepsy.

• Trouble hearing.

• Trouble with vision and changes in eye movements.

• Pain or trouble feeling sensations such as touch.

• Bladder and bowel issues, including constipation and urinary incontinence.

• Mental health conditions, such as emotional conditions and behavior issues.

The brain condition causing cerebral palsy doesn't change with time. Symptoms usually don't worsen with age. However, as the child gets older, some symptoms might become more or less clear. And muscle shortening and muscle rigidity can worsen if not treated aggressively.

When to see a doctor

Contact your child's health care professional and get a prompt diagnosis if your child has symptoms of a movement condition. Also see a health professional if your child has delays in development.

See your child's health care professional if you have concerns about episodes of loss of awareness or of irregular bodily movements or posture. It's also important to contact your child's health care professional if your child has trouble swallowing, poor coordination, eye muscle imbalance or other developmental issues.

Causes

Cerebral palsy is caused by irregular brain development or damage to the developing brain. This usually happens before a child is born, but it can occur at birth or in early infancy. Often the cause isn't known. Many factors can lead to changes in brain development. Some include:

• Gene changes that result in genetic conditions or differences in brain development.

• Maternal infections that affect an unborn baby.

• Stroke, which interrupts blood supply to the developing brain.

• Bleeding into the brain in the womb or as a newborn.

• Infant infections that cause swelling in or around the brain.

• Traumatic head injury to an infant, such as from a motor vehicle accident, fall or physical trauma.

• Lack of oxygen to the brain related to a hard labor or delivery, although this cause is less common than previously thought.

Risk factors

A number of factors are associated with an increased risk of cerebral palsy.

Maternal health

Certain infections or toxic exposures during pregnancy can significantly increase cerebral palsy risk to the baby. Inflammation triggered by infection or fever can damage the unborn baby's developing brain.

• Cytomegalovirus. This common virus causes flu-like symptoms. If a mother has her first active infection during pregnancy, it can lead to birth defects.

• German measles, known as rubella. This viral infection can be prevented with a vaccine.

• Herpes. This infection can be passed from mother to child during pregnancy, affecting the womb and placenta.

• Syphilis. This is a bacterial infection that's usually spread by sexual contact.

• Toxoplasmosis. This infection is caused by a parasite found in contaminated food, soil and the feces of infected cats.

• Zika virus infection. This infection is spread through mosquito bites and can affect the brain development of an unborn baby.

• Intrauterine infections. This includes infections of the placenta or fetal membranes.

• Exposure to toxins. One example is exposure to methyl mercury.

• Other conditions. Other conditions affecting the mother that can slightly increase the risk of cerebral palsy include thyroid conditions, preeclampsia or seizures.

Infant illness

Illnesses in a newborn baby that can greatly increase the risk of cerebral palsy include:

• Bacterial meningitis. This bacterial infection causes swelling in the membranes surrounding the brain and spinal cord.

• Viral encephalitis. This viral infection also causes swelling in the membranes surrounding the brain and spinal cord.

• Severe or untreated jaundice. Jaundice appears as a yellowing of the skin and eyes. The condition occurs when certain byproducts of "used" blood cells aren't filtered from the bloodstream.

• Bleeding into the brain. This condition is commonly caused by the baby having a stroke in the womb or in early infancy.

Factors of pregnancy and birth

The potential contribution from each is limited, but these pregnancy and birth factors may increase the risk of cerebral palsy risk:

• Low birth weight. Babies who weigh less than 5.5 pounds (2.5 kilograms) are at higher risk of developing cerebral palsy. This risk increases as birth weight drops.

• Multiple babies. Cerebral palsy risk increases with the number of babies sharing the uterus. The risk also can be related to the likelihood of premature birth and low birth weight. If one or more of the babies die, the survivors' risk of cerebral palsy increases.

• Premature birth. Babies born prematurely are at higher risk of cerebral palsy. The earlier a baby is born, the greater the cerebral palsy risk.

• Delivery complications. Events during labor and delivery may increase the risk of cerebral palsy.

Complications

Muscle weakness, muscle spasticity and trouble with coordination can contribute to complications in childhood or in adulthood, including:

• Contracture. Contracture is muscle tissue shortening due to severe muscle tightening. This can be the result of spasticity. Contracture can slow bone growth, cause bones to bend, and result in joint changes, dislocation or partial dislocation. These can include a dislocated hip, a curved spine or other bone changes.

• Malnutrition. Trouble with swallowing and feeding can make it hard to get enough nutrition, particularly for an infant. This can impair growth and weaken bones. Some children or adults need a feeding tube to get enough nutrition.

• Mental health conditions. People with cerebral palsy might have mental health conditions, such as depression. Social isolation and the challenges of coping with disabilities can contribute to depression. Behavior issues also can occur.

• Heart and lung disease. People with cerebral palsy may develop heart disease, lung disease and breathing conditions. Trouble swallowing can result in respiratory issues, such as aspiration pneumonia. Aspiration pneumonia happens when a child inhales food, drink, saliva or vomit into the lungs.

• Osteoarthritis. Pressure on joints or misalignment of joints from muscle spasticity may lead to this painful bone disease.

• Osteoporosis. Fractures due to low bone density can result from lack of mobility, poor nutrition and anti-seizure medicines.

• Other complications. These can include sleep conditions, chronic pain, skin breakdown, intestinal issues and issues with oral health.

Prevention

Often cerebral palsy can't be prevented, but you can reduce risks. If you're pregnant or planning to become pregnant, take these steps to minimize pregnancy complications:

• Make sure you're vaccinated. Getting vaccinated against diseases such as rubella might prevent an infection. It's best to make sure you're fully vaccinated before getting pregnant.

• Take care of yourself. The healthier you are heading into a pregnancy, the less likely you'll be to develop an infection that results in cerebral palsy.

• Seek early and continuous prenatal care.See your health care professional regularly during pregnancy. Proper prenatal care can reduce health risks to you and your unborn baby. Seeing your health care professional regularly can help prevent premature birth, low birth weight and infections.

• Avoid alcohol, tobacco and illegal drugs.These have been linked to cerebral palsy risk.

Rarely, cerebral palsy can be caused by brain damage that occurs in childhood. Practice good general safety. Prevent head injuries by providing your child with a car seat, bicycle helmet, safety rails on the bed and appropriate supervision.

Managing and Treating Cerebral Palsy

There is no cure for cerebral palsy, but with the right treatments and interventions, children with CP can lead fulfilling lives:

- Therapies: Physical, occupational, and speech therapies are essential for improving mobility, coordination, and communication skills. Early intervention is crucial.

- Assistive Devices: Mobility aids such as braces,

wheelchairs, and communication devices can greatly enhance a child's independence.

- Medical Interventions: Medications to manage spasticity, surgeries to correct joint issues, and treatments to address associated conditions like seizures can help improve quality of life.

Supporting a Child with Cerebral Palsy

Raising a child with Cerebral Palsy requires patience, love, and dedication. Here are some tips for parents and caregivers:

- Focus on Abilities, Not Disabilities: Celebrate your child's achievements, no matter how small. Encourage their strengths and help them build self-confidence.

- Stay Informed and Proactive: Learn as much as you can about Cerebral Palsy and advocate for your child's needs. Regular medical checkups and continuous therapy can prevent complications and improve outcomes.

- Join Support Networks: Connecting with other parents of children with CP can provide valuable emotional support and practical advice.

Prevention and Awareness

While not all cases of cerebral palsy can be prevented, certain precautions can reduce the risk:

- Prenatal Care: Regular checkups during pregnancy,

vaccinations against infections like rubella, and avoiding alcohol, tobacco, and drugs can minimize risks.

- Safety Measures: Protecting your child from head injuries through the use of car seats, helmets, and proper supervision can prevent brain damage after birth.

Conclusion

Cerebral palsy presents unique challenges, but with the right care and support, children with Cerebral Palsy can thrive. By understanding the condition and seeking early interventions, parents can help their children lead happy, fulfilling lives.

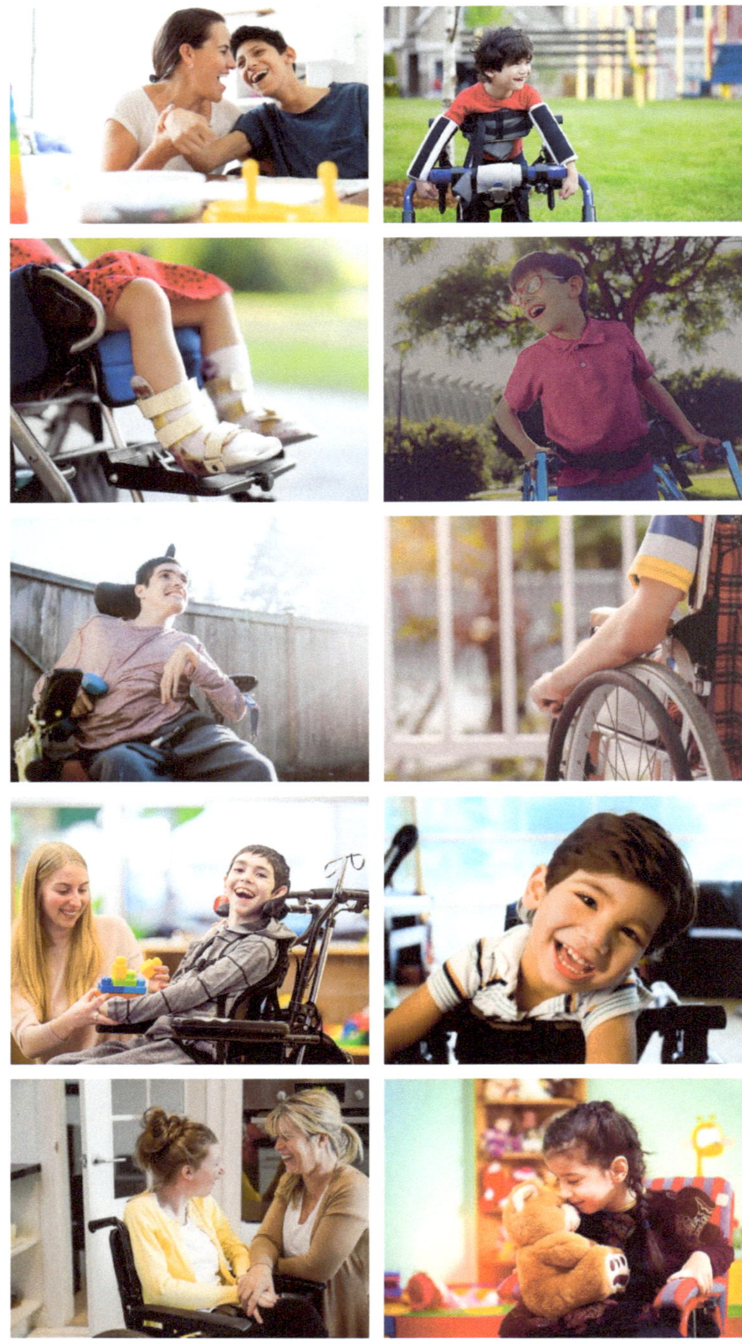

HOW TO HELP SPECIAL NEEDS CHILDREN ACHIEVE THEIR GOALS

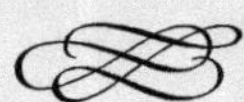

Set goals

• Work with your child to set goals they want to work toward. Find out what they are interested in and what they want to achieve. Even if your child is non-verbal, you can use their body language and responses, and progress in therapy to help set goals to work on. This also provides more motivation and incentive for your child because they are working toward something they find meaningful.

Celebrate achievements

• We often measure success by the big milestones in life, first steps, first words, first day of school. However, for a child with special needs, those milestones might look different.

Celebrating both the small and big victories helps reinforce positive development and can play a significant role in boosting your child's self-esteem.

Collaborate with teachers and therapists

• Talk about ways that you can work together to create consistency in building skills and fostering independence. Open communication allows you to share strategies that are or aren't working well and come up with new approaches so you are all on the same page.

Listen and Support

• We listen to children with special needs because;

• It acknowledges their right to be listened to and for their views and experiences to be taken seriously about matters that affect them and we also listen to special needs children to make a difference on how they feel about themselves. Children with special needs need more support, someone to look up to. Together we can make a difference in their lives.

Promote Independence

• Raising a child with special needs can be a lot of work. You want to provide them with the best support and services to maximize their potential while protecting them from being hurt. Depending on the nature of your child's needs, you may become over protective in an effort to help them be more successful. It is important to build your child's confidence and independence so they realize how much they can do on their own.

Their special needs don't have to hold them back.

Provide choices

• One easy way of starting to build independence is by giving your child choices so they are more in control of their life. This can be applied to so many situations whether it's deciding between wearing a blue shirt or a green shirt, picking a banana or an orange for snack or choosing whether to brush their teeth or put on pyjamas first.

They are able to advocate for their preferences.

Avoid doing things for them

• If your child is capable of brushing their own hair or getting dressed by themselves, let them do it, even if it means allowing for extra time. It might be easier for you to do it for them, but it doesn't help them in the long run. If a task takes a while, keep giving them opportunities to practice and improve their skills.

Provide challenges

• Don't make everything just easy just so your child will succeed. Be strategic in giving them challenges that they can achieve with some effort or practice. They will begin to see that they can do things if they put their mind to it and work hard. If a task is a struggle for them, consider ways to adopt it to their current abilities. As they develop their skills, you can continue to make adjustments to build their independence.

Use assistive devices as appropriate

• Whether it's a communication device, special utensils, buttons and switches, or some technology, find what works for your child. These devices are designed to support them and help them to be more successful and independent. Learn how to use assistive technology to benefit their development and help them become more accustomed to how to use it.

ABUSE AND NEGLECT IN SPECIAL NEEDS CHILDREN

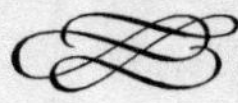

Children with special needs are nearly four times more likely to be physically abused or neglected and more than three times more likely to be sexually abused when compared to children without special needs.

Special needs children are also victims of bullying. Corporal punishment, and other types of maltreatment at the hands of the other students and teachers at school and most of special needs children, the majority of abusers are family members, relatives, caregivers, neighbors, classmates, educators or staff members assigned to support the child with special needs that's why it's very important to have a loving heart to care for children or individuals with special needs.

It takes courage, patience and understanding to take care of children or individuals with special needs.

And I would like to advise parents, caregivers and providers to take abuse and neglect class to understand more of their rights and to always have integrity in everything you do and to remind parents to always advocate for their children no matter what.

It could be your daughter, son, brother, sister, uncle, aunt, mother, father, cousin, niece, nephew, grandmother, grandfather, friend, neighbor, never stop loving them, caring for them, listening to them and cheering them up. They didn't choose who they became and what they go through.

They are human beings and that's why they deserve advocacy and to be treated right.

At the end of this book, I will share with you some of the pictures of the children with special needs in our program in Rwanda who don't have any support, resources, clothes, diapers who don't even have access to Education, healthcare and good nutrition and if you are a parent of special needs child in USA, Canada, Europe, Australia and some other developed countries in Asia please be grateful that at least your child has support and know that these parents are struggling a lot, they wish they can be in your position. Their wish is to one day be recognized and be able to get some support from the government as well so they can take good care of their children.

This book is going to help so many parents with special needs around the World. Guardians and some providers on some tips on how to raise on how to raise a successful special need child.

Whoever will be touched by these children please go to our website and select the child you would like to support and God will bless you.

A message from Diana Uwera, the CEO and Founder of International Community Center and the author of this book on how children should be treated in Africa.

I am an advocate for human rights, I advocate for children with special needs, single mothers, domestic violence survivors, men who are abused by women, girls and boys who are rape victims but this book is for special needs children and this book is so special because it's my first book and more books are coming.

I started working with special needs children in 2015 in the United States of America as a host home provider for children with special needs with my wonderful agency called Mosaic Agency that works with people with special needs and from then I never stopped caring for people with special needs.

As a provider, I took so many trainings that helped me pursue my purpose in life.

I had a call to care for humanity and that made it easier to bond with people with special needs. I still take care of them and they are part of my family. It takes courage and patience and to build trust in them by loving and caring for them. Sometimes you have to make it fun with full of positivity to make it easier for you as a provider. In 2022 I traveled to Rwanda in Africa , I decided to gather parents who have special needs children to support them emotionally by talking to them and giving them words of encouragement and to encourage them not to give up and financially to be able to buy diapers, food and be able to provide some basic needs. We are more blessed in blessing others. They are so grateful for everything we do for them and I am inviting anyone who want to join the cause to feel free to join and transform someone's life.

We lost one young mother of one of our special needs children in 2023 and it was a sudden death. I was a blessing to her before she passed away and I will be forever grateful to see that I was able to touch her life in just one year and her child is still in our program and she is doing great.

She left one young beautiful girl with cerebral palsy who needs full time caregiver. We are still following up with that child and supporting her. It's the promise that I made to myself to keep supporting that child because her mother believed in me.

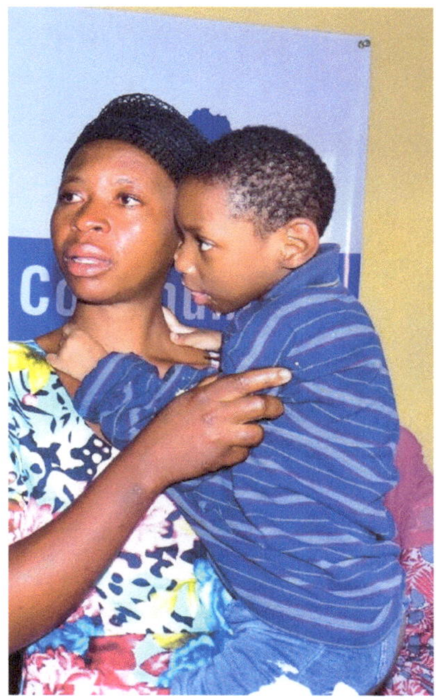

Died in 2023 and left a child with special needs. May her soul rest in peace. International Community Center is attending the care of the child. Special thanks to Mr. Larry who helps this child to get basic needs. We need more people like Larry.

My wish is to one day see a special need child in Africa being taken care of and for the parents of special needs children to have a support system where they don't have to worry about leaving their children unattended to step out of the house to find food and other necessities because they don't have any sort of support.

Most of mothers of special needs children are single mothers because their husbands left them the moment they saw a special need child; the community is against those mothers and most of them do labor jobs on daily basis for survival. They are forced to lock their special needs children in the house unattended for approximately six hours to be able to feed them and afford diapers and pads for those who have teenager girls. They have to work to get their children medication as well.

These women do labor jobs, washing clothes for people and some of them sell tomatoes or bananas on the streets.

As an advocate for human rights, I want my voice to be heard for an African child with special needs.

No child should be locked home alone unattended especially those who can't move or walk or speak. Imagine how they starve until their mothers return back. Anything can happen in those six hours.

RIGHTS AND RESPONSIBILITIES

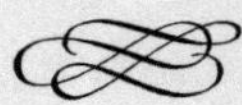

The government should promote the development of all children with special needs and realize their rights and give them access to basic needs because parents of children with special needs face a lot of challenges that includes healthcare for their well-being, access to the right medication, educational facilities, Speech therapists, Counsellors, Special Education Teachers, Sign Language Teachers, Diapers, Special diet. Every parent deserves allowance to help their children with special needs without worrying too much about everything and together we can make a difference in a special needs child's life.

Diana Uwera is a single mother of three wonderful boys, she knows the sacrifice of being a single mother especially in Africa.

That's why she gathered these wonderful mothers of children with special needs in Rwanda and encouraged them to create a support group where they meet once a month and support each other, share the achievements they made and it really helps them a lot.

They listen to each other, encourage each other, meet with all their children, sometimes we send our ICC supporting team to join them and talk to them and give them an envelope with some money to help them buy some basic needs, words of encouragement and hope and they leave everyone happy.

Together we can change lives by supporting a special needs child.

The Power of Advocacy and Collective Voice

As parents of children with special needs, we often find ourselves facing monumental challenges—challenges that can feel isolating, overwhelming, and insurmountable. But one of the most powerful tools at our disposal is our collective voice. When we come together as a community of parents, caregivers, and advocates, our ability to create change multiplies.

Advocacy is not just about speaking up for your own child; it's about standing together to ensure that all children with special needs are seen, heard, and supported. It's about demanding that our governments, institutions, and societies recognize the value and potential of every child, regardless of their abilities.

In many African countries, the resources and support systems for children with special needs are severely lacking. Parents are often left to navigate these challenges alone, without the necessary tools or assistance. But when we unite and advocate as a collective, we can amplify our message and push for the systemic changes that are so desperately needed.

Imagine the impact if every parent, every caregiver, every teacher, and every community member raised their voice to demand better services, inclusive education, and equitable opportunities for our children. Together, we can challenge the status quo and push for policies that reflect the needs and rights of children with special needs.

Advocacy is also about raising awareness. By sharing our stories and experiences, we educate others and dismantle the misconceptions and stigmas that often surround special needs. Every time we speak out, we not only advocate for our children but also for future generations of children with special needs, paving the way for a more inclusive and compassionate society.

But advocacy is not a solo endeavor. It thrives on community. It grows stronger when we support one another, share resources, and collaborate towards common goals. When parents unite, we become a formidable force, capable of driving change not just within our own families, but within our communities and beyond.

This book, "I Am Your Gift," is not just a guide for raising children with special needs; it is a call to action. It is an invitation to join a movement that seeks to transform the way our societies view and treat children with special needs. Let this book inspire you to become an advocate— not just for your child, but for all children with special needs. Let it remind you that you are not alone in this journey, and that together, our collective voice can—and will—make a difference.

The Inherent Value of Every Child

Every child is a gift, a unique and irreplaceable treasure with their own inherent worth, potential, and beauty. This is a truth that stands firm regardless of a child's abilities, challenges, or the labels society may place upon them. In a world that often measures worth by conventional standards of success and ability, it is vital to remember and proclaim that the value of a child is not diminished by their special needs—in fact, it is often enriched by the perspectives, strengths, and insights they bring to our lives.

Children with special needs teach us invaluable lessons about patience, resilience, and unconditional love. They show us the beauty of different ways of being and interacting with the world. These children challenge the limitations of our own understanding and expand our capacity for empathy, compassion, and acceptance.

In African cultures, and indeed across the world, there is a pressing need to shift our perceptions—to see beyond the special needs to the individual, to recognize that every child, regardless of their abilities, has something precious to offer. They may communicate in ways that are different, achieve milestones at their own pace, and express themselves uniquely, but these differences do not lessen their value. Rather, they add to the rich tapestry of human experience.

We must learn to see the gifts within each child, not despite their challenges but through them. Every child deserves to be seen, celebrated, and supported in a way that honors their individuality. This means providing them with the love, education, and opportunities they need to thrive. It means advocating for a society that does not merely tolerate differences but embraces them, recognizing that diversity in ability enriches us all.

To the parents reading this book, know that your child is not a burden, but a blessing. The journey may be difficult, and the road may be long, but the value of your child is immeasurable. By nurturing their strengths, supporting their needs, and advocating for their rights, you affirm their worth not just in your own life, but in the world at large.

In a society that too often fails to see the potential in every child, let this book be a reminder and a call to action: every child has value. Every child deserves to be seen for who they truly are—a gift to be cherished, nurtured, and celebrated.

The Crucial Role of Education and Awareness

Education and awareness are the cornerstones of understanding, acceptance, and inclusion for children with special needs. In many societies, especially in African countries, a lack of knowledge about special needs often leads to fear, stigma, and exclusion. But through education and raising awareness, we can transform these negative perceptions into a culture of empathy, support, and inclusion.

Education is not just about teaching children with special needs; it's also about educating parents, teachers, communities, and policymakers. When people are informed about the nature of different special needs, they are better equipped to provide the necessary support and accommodations. Understanding the specific challenges and strengths of children with special needs allows for the creation of learning environments that nurture their potential and enable them to thrive.

For parents, education begins with understanding their

child's unique needs. It involves learning about the specific special needs, recognizing the symptoms, and knowing how to support their child's development. This knowledge empowers parents to be strong advocates for their children, ensuring they receive the appropriate interventions and services that can make a significant difference in their lives.

For teachers and educators, awareness is key to fostering an inclusive classroom where all students can learn and grow together. Teachers who are educated about special needs can modify their teaching strategies to accommodate diverse learning styles and needs, creating a supportive environment where every child can succeed. This not only benefits children with special needs but enriches the educational experience for all students, promoting values of empathy, diversity, and mutual respect.

Raising awareness within the broader community is equally important. When communities are educated about the realities of living with a special need, they are more likely to support inclusive policies, provide necessary resources, and create environments where children with special needs are welcomed and valued. Awareness campaigns can dispel myths, reduce stigma, and foster a sense of collective responsibility towards ensuring that all children have the opportunity to reach their full potential.

Moreover, education and awareness extend to policymakers and government officials. When those in positions of power are informed about the challenges faced by children with special needs and their families, they are more likely to implement policies that provide the necessary support, such as access to special education services, healthcare, and social support systems. Advocacy for better education and awareness at the governmental level can lead to systemic changes that benefit not only individual children but society as a whole.

In "I Am Your Gift," I aim to shed light on the importance of education and awareness in transforming the lives of children with special needs. It is through understanding and knowledge that we can build a world where these children are not just accommodated, but celebrated for the unique gifts they bring to our lives. By educating ourselves and others, we take the first steps toward creating a more inclusive, supportive, and compassionate world for all children.

Inspiring Hope and Resilience

Raising a child with special needs is a journey filled with unique challenges, moments of uncertainty, and often, a sense of isolation. But it is also a journey marked by profound love, unexpected joy, and the incredible strength that both you and your child possess. In the face of adversity, it is hope and resilience that will guide you through the darkest days and illuminate the path ahead.

Hope is the belief that no matter how difficult today may be, tomorrow holds the promise of something better. It is the quiet assurance that your child has the capacity to grow, learn, and thrive, even in the face of obstacles. Hope is what keeps you moving forward, pushing past the fear and doubt, and believing in the possibilities that lie within your child.

As you navigate this journey, it's important to recognize that resilience is not about never feeling discouraged or overwhelmed. Rather, resilience is the ability to rise each time you are knocked down. It's the courage to face each challenge head-on, armed with the knowledge that every setback is an opportunity to grow stronger and wiser.

Resilience is not only found in parents but in children as well. Children with special needs often display a remarkable ability to adapt, learn, and flourish despite the difficulties they encounter. They teach us that resilience is not just about enduring hardships but about finding ways to overcome them with grace and determination. Every milestone they reach, every new skill they acquire, is a testament to their inner strength and tenacity.

In "I Am Your Gift," I want to remind you that it's okay to have moments of doubt or exhaustion. What matters most is that you continue to believe in your child and in yourself. Remember that you are not alone on this journey—there are countless parents who share your struggles, and together, you form a community of resilience and hope.

Let the stories of others who have walked this path before you serve as beacons of hope. They have faced the same fears, encountered similar obstacles, and yet, they have persevered. Their experiences show that while the road may be difficult, it is also filled with moments of profound joy, pride, and love.

Allow yourself to be inspired by the progress your child makes, no matter how small it may seem. Each step forward, each new achievement, is a victory worth celebrating. These moments are reminders that your efforts are making a difference, that your love and support are helping your child to thrive.

Ultimately, this journey is about more than just overcoming challenges—it's about discovering the depth of your own resilience and the boundless potential within your child. It's about finding hope in the most unexpected places and realizing that you are stronger and more capable than you ever imagined.

As you continue on this path, hold onto hope as your guiding star. Nurture resilience in yourself and in your child, knowing that together, you can face whatever challenges come your way. And always remember: you are not alone, and your journey, while difficult, is also filled with the possibility of joy, growth, and the enduring power of love.

A Call for Government Responsibility and Social Justice

As a parent of a child with special needs, you understand the daily challenges, triumphs, and heartaches that come with this journey. You are your child's greatest advocate, their fiercest protector, and their most steadfast supporter. But despite your unwavering dedication, there are limits to what you can achieve alone. This is where the responsibility of government and the pursuit of social justice must come into play.

In many African countries, and indeed around the world, children with special needs and their families are often overlooked, marginalized, and denied the resources they desperately need. This neglect is not just an oversight—it is a profound injustice. It is time for our governments to acknowledge their role in perpetuating these inequalities and to take decisive action to correct them.

Government responsibility is not a matter of charity; it is a matter of rights. Every child, regardless of their abilities, has the right to access education, healthcare, and social services that allow them to live a life of dignity and opportunity. It is the duty of our governments to ensure that these rights are upheld. Yet, too often, families are left to fend for themselves, struggling to navigate a system that fails to provide even the most basic support.

I am raising my voice, and I urge you to raise yours, to demand that our leaders do better. Governments must allocate the necessary resources to support children with special needs and their families. This includes funding for special education programs, access to specialized healthcare, and the creation of social services that provide respite and support for parents. Policies must be enacted and enforced to protect the rights of children with special needs, ensuring that they are not only included but also celebrated within our societies.

Social justice for children with special needs is about more than just access to resources; it is about changing the very fabric of our societies. It is about dismantling the stigma and discrimination that have kept these children in the shadows for far too long. It is about creating a world where every child is valued for who they are, not overlooked because of what they are perceived to lack.

This is a call to action for all of us—not just parents, but educators, healthcare providers, community leaders, and citizens. We must hold our governments accountable and push for policies that reflect our collective commitment to equality and inclusion. We must demand that our societies recognize the worth of every child and provide the necessary support to help them reach their full potential.

To the governments of African nations and beyond: the time for inaction has passed. The future of our children is at stake, and with it, the future of our societies. We cannot claim to be just or equitable if we continue to neglect those who need us the most. It is your responsibility to create the frameworks, provide the funding, and enforce the laws that will ensure every child with special needs can thrive.

To my fellow parents and advocates: let our voices be heard. Together, we can be a force for change, a collective voice that demands justice, equity, and dignity for our children. We owe it to our children to fight for a world where they are not just accepted, but embraced and supported in all their uniqueness.

I Am Your Gift is not just a book—it is a movement. A movement that calls for government responsibility, social justice, and a brighter, more inclusive future for all children. Let us stand together and make this vision a reality.

A Vision for the Future

As we journey through the complexities of raising children with special needs, it's important to hold on to a vision of what the future can—and should—be. This vision is not just a dream; it is a goal, a promise to our children, and a commitment to building a world where they are fully included, supported, and celebrated for who they are.

I envision a future where every child with special needs is given the opportunity to thrive. In this future, our societies will be built on a foundation of inclusion, where differences are not just accepted but valued. Schools will be places of learning for all children, with teachers trained to recognize and nurture the potential in every student, regardless of their abilities. No longer will children with special needs be sidelined or excluded; instead, they will learn alongside their peers, contributing their unique perspectives and strengths.

In this future, healthcare systems will be fully equipped to meet the needs of every child. Specialized care will be accessible to all, not just those who can afford it. Early intervention programs will be readily available, ensuring that every child has the best start in life. Parents will have the support they need, including access to therapies, medical care, and resources that empower them to care for their children without being overwhelmed by the financial and emotional burdens.

Communities will be strongholds of support and understanding. In this future, no family will have to face the challenges of raising a child with special needs alone. There will be networks of support, both formal and informal, where parents can find guidance, respite, and camaraderie. Public spaces, from playgrounds to workplaces, will be designed with accessibility in mind, ensuring that everyone can participate fully in community life.

Our governments will take active responsibility for ensuring the rights of all children are upheld. Policies will be crafted with the input of those who are directly affected, and resources will be allocated to ensure that every child with special needs has access to education, healthcare, and social services. Laws will be enforced to protect against discrimination, and there will be accountability at every level of government to ensure that these protections are not just words on paper, but realities in the lives of our children.

Most importantly, I envision a future where the stigma surrounding special needs has been eradicated. In this future, awareness and education will have paved the way for a culture of empathy and respect. Children with special needs will no longer be seen as 'different' or 'less than,' but as individuals with their own gifts, capable of contributing to society in meaningful ways. Our world will be richer for the diversity of abilities and experiences, and we will all be better for it.

This is the future I see—a future where every child, regardless of their needs, is given the chance to shine. It is a future that we must work toward together, as parents, educators, advocates, and citizens. The path may be long, and the challenges great, but this vision is within our reach. With determination, compassion, and collective action, we can make this future a reality for our children.

Let "I Am Your Gift" be a beacon of hope and a call to action. Together, we can build a world where every child is valued, every family is supported, and every society is enriched by the contributions of its most vulnerable members. This is the future we owe to our children, and it is a future worth fighting for.

The Importance of Self-Care and Community Support

As a parent of a child with special needs, you give so much of yourself every day—your time, energy, love, and patience. Your dedication to your child is unwavering, and your resilience is remarkable. But in the midst of caring for your child, it's easy to forget something very important: you must also care for yourself.

Self-care is not a luxury; it is a necessity. It is essential to your well-being and your ability to continue being the loving, supportive parent your child needs. Taking time for yourself is not selfish; it is an act of strength. It allows you to recharge, to maintain your health, both physically and mentally, and to be present for your child in the best possible way.

Self-care can take many forms. It might be as simple as a few moments of quiet reflection in the morning, a walk in nature, or a chat with a friend who understands. It could be finding time for a hobby you enjoy, seeking professional support when you need it, or simply allowing yourself to rest without guilt. Whatever self-care looks like for you, it's crucial to make it a regular part of your life.

But self-care doesn't happen in isolation. It is deeply connected to the support systems we build around ourselves. This is where community comes in. Community support is vital for parents of children with special needs. The journey you are on can be overwhelming, and it is not one you should have to face alone. Surrounding yourself with a network of people who understand and can offer help, whether it's emotional support, practical assistance, or just someone to listen, can make a world of difference.

Seek out other parents who are walking a similar path. Join support groups, whether in person or online, where you can share experiences, exchange advice, and find encouragement. Building a community of support can provide you with a sense of belonging and the reassurance that you are not alone in your struggles or your joys.

In addition to connecting with other parents, reach out to family, friends, and neighbors who can offer their support. Don't hesitate to ask for help when you need it —whether it's someone to watch your child for a few hours, help with household chores, or simply provide a listening ear. People often want to help but don't know how; by reaching out, you give them the opportunity to support you and your child.

Remember, your well-being is just as important as your child's. By taking care of yourself, you are better equipped to care for your child. You'll find that when you are rested, supported, and emotionally healthy, you are more patient, more present, and more capable of meeting your child's needs.

Finally, know that it's okay to feel vulnerable, to have moments of doubt, and to seek out support. No one has all the answers, and there is no one 'right' way to navigate this journey. What matters is that you take care of yourself, lean on your community, and continue to show up with love and resilience for your child.

In "I Am Your Gift," I want to remind you that you are not just a caregiver—you are also a person with your own needs, dreams, and emotions. Embracing self-care and seeking community support are vital steps in maintaining your strength and well-being. You are doing an incredible job, and by caring for yourself, you are ensuring that you can continue to be the amazing parent your child needs.

A CALL TO COMPASSION

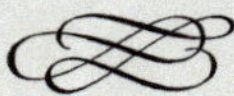

Here are some pictures of our beautiful children and staff at our centre.

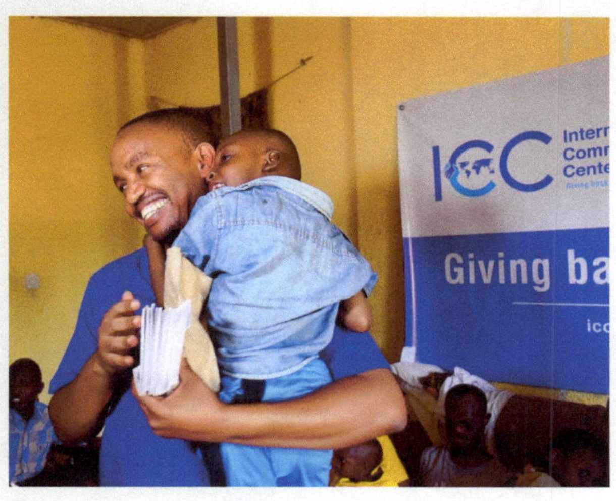

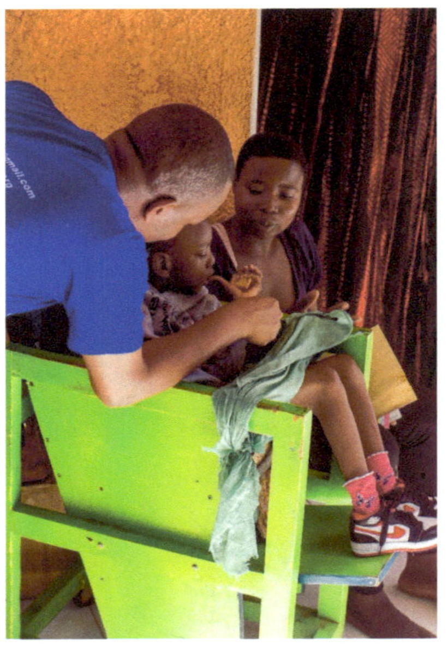

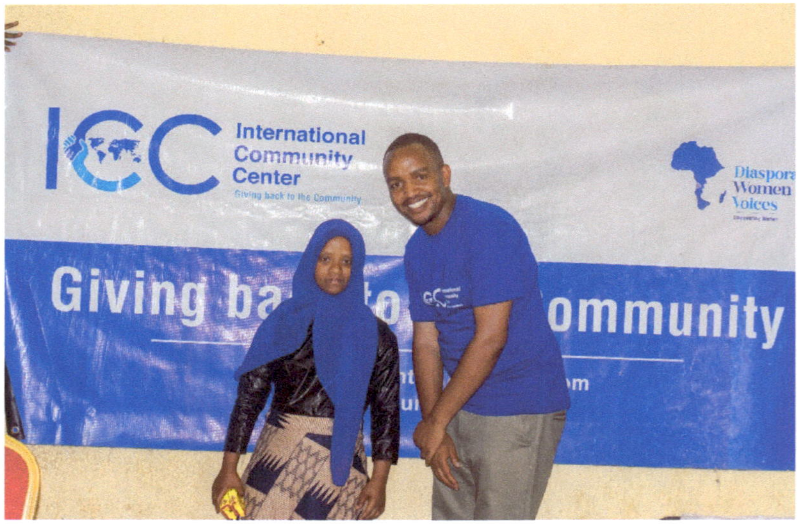
ICC
International
Community
Center
Giving back to the Community
Giving ba   o   ommunity
Diaspora
Women
Voices

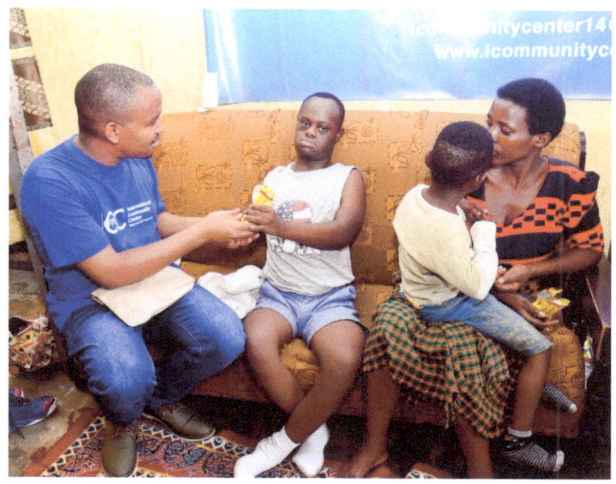

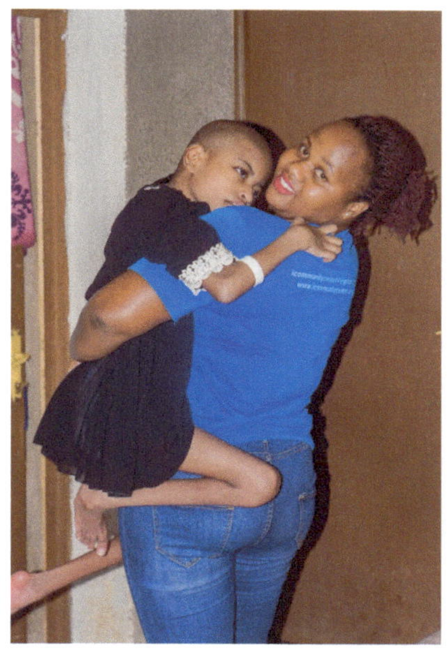

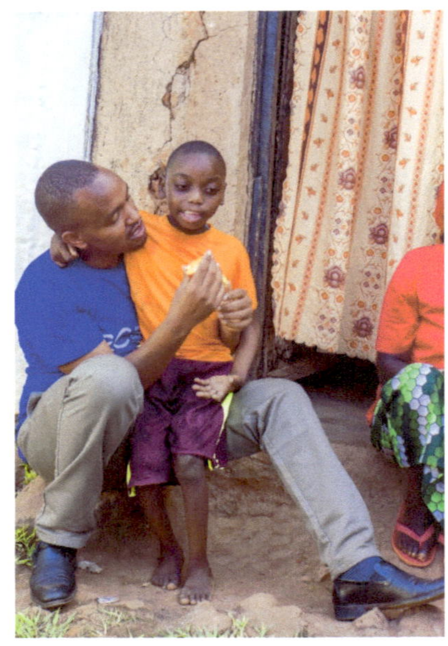

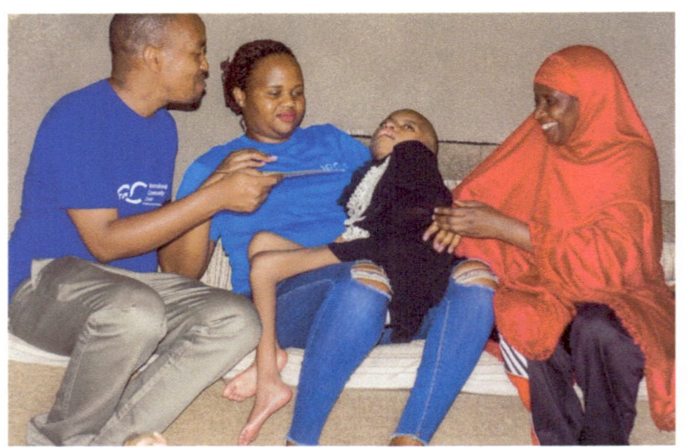

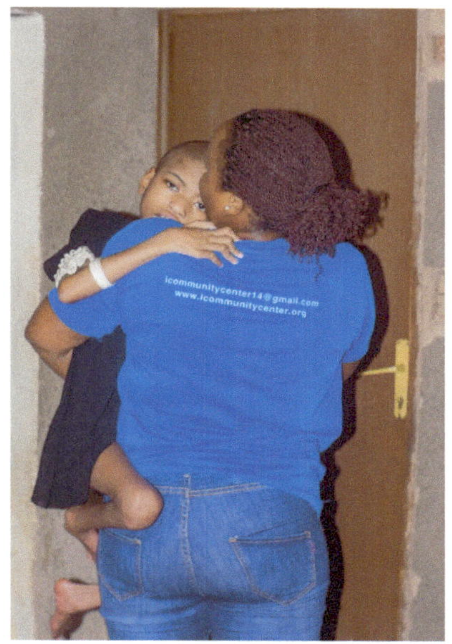
icommunitycenter14@gmail.com
www.icommunitycenter.org

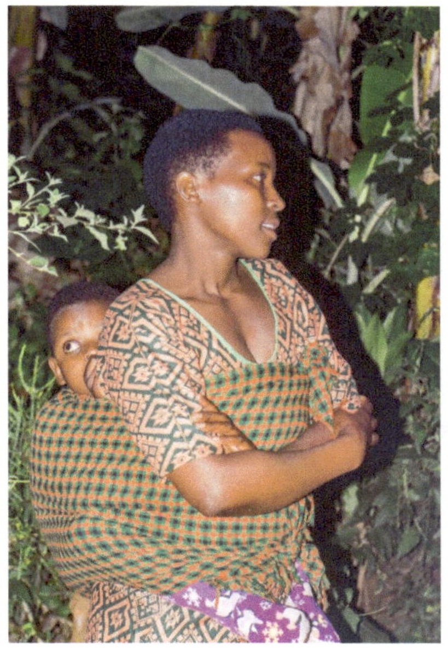

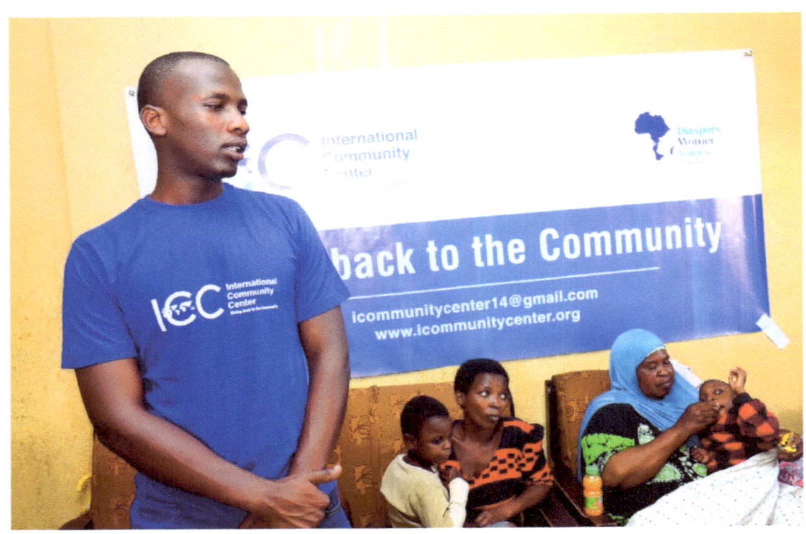
International
Community
Center
back to the Community
icommunitycenter14@gmail.com
www.icommunitycenter.org

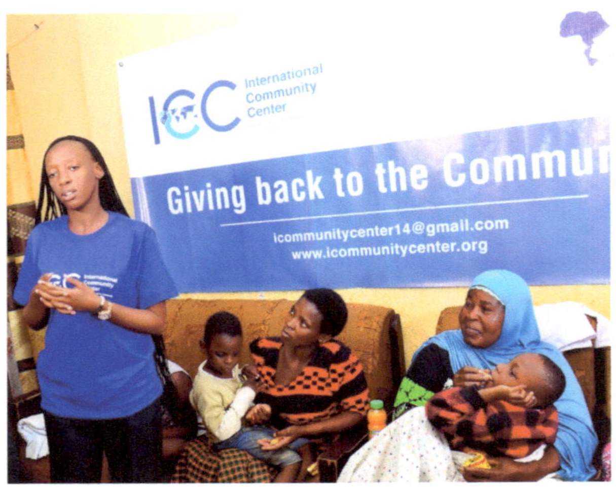
ICC International
Community
Center
Giving back to the Commur
icommunitycenter14@gmail.com
www.icommunitycenter.org

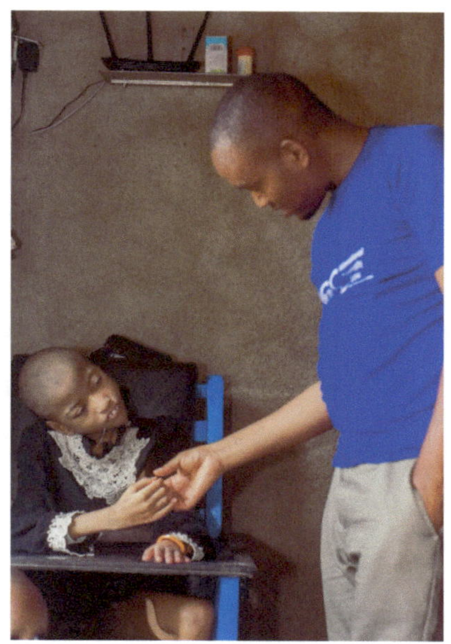

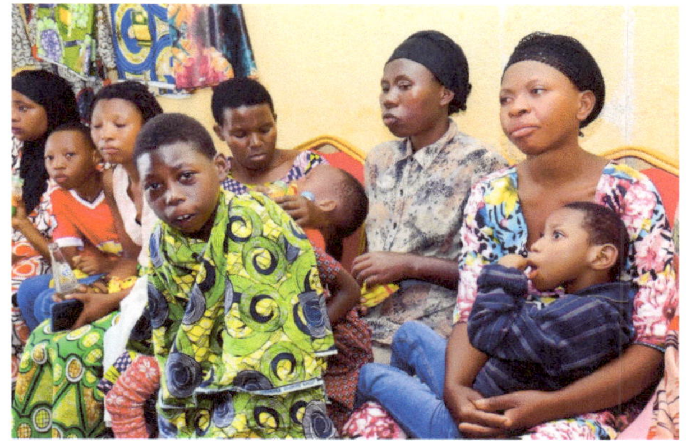

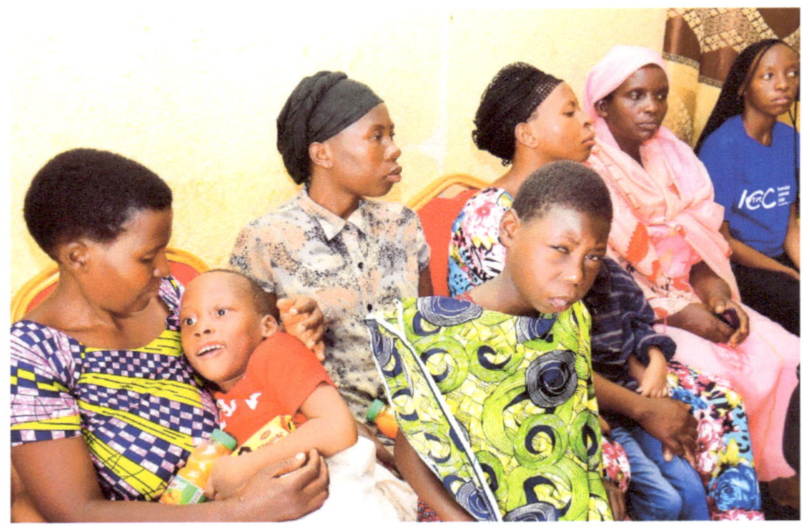

MESSAGES FROM MY SONS

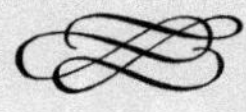

Diana's three sons have something to say

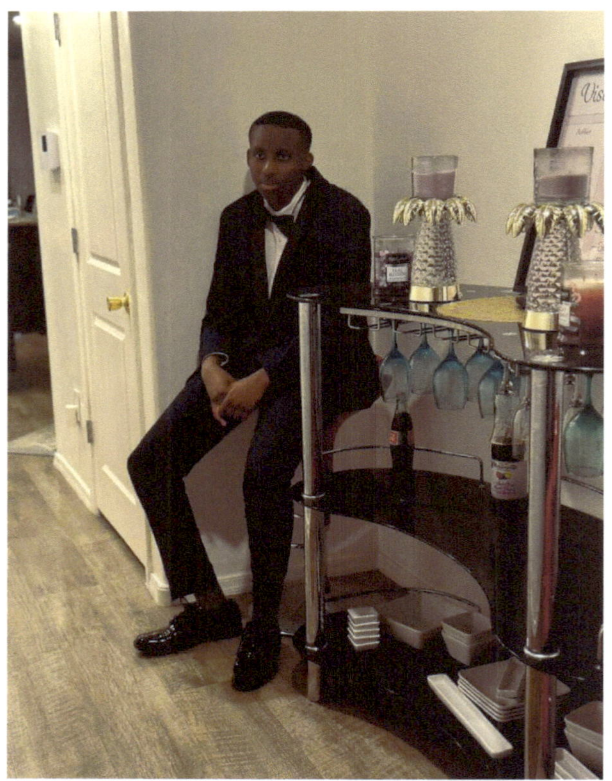

Derrick

Derrick's Message to His Mom Diana

"Mom, I want to thank you a million times for everything you're doing to advocate for children with special needs. You've gone so many extra miles to help these kids, and your dedication is truly inspiring. I see how hard you work and how much you care, and I'm so proud to be your son.

To all the parents out there who are raising children with special needs: please, never give up. I know it's tough, and there are days when it feels like the challenges are too great, but you're not alone. Keep going, keep fighting, and know that your efforts make a world of difference. Your love and support mean everything to your child, just like my mom's love and support mean the world to me. Together, we can create a better future for all our children."

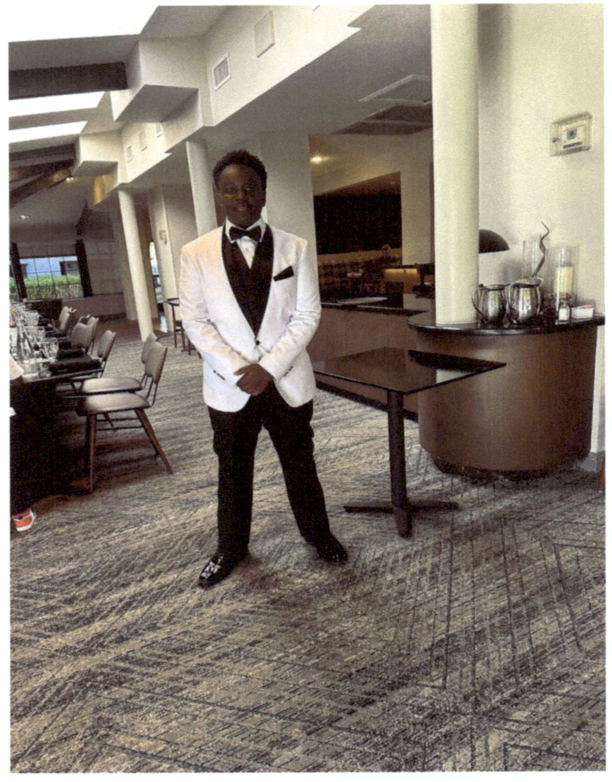

Brian

Brian Junior's Message to His Mom Diana

"When I see how much I have—so many pairs of shoes, clothes, and food—I can't help but think of the children who have nothing. It makes me thank God so much for what I have.

Mom, thank you for taking care of children in need, especially those with special needs. I've learned so much from you about loving and caring for people who need it the most. I'm so proud to be your son, and I hope I can be as kind and giving as you are."

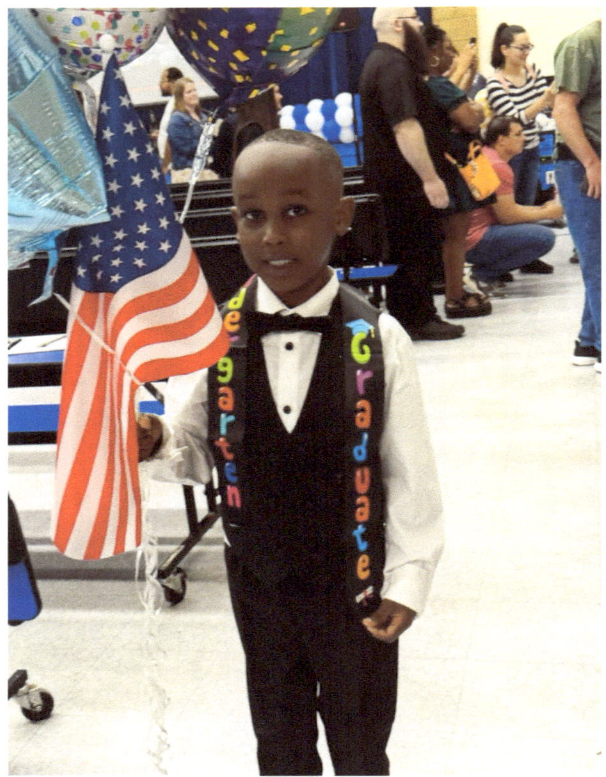

Prince

Prince's Message to His Mom Diana

"Mom, the video I watched made me cry when I saw a child moving on his tummy in the dirt. I cried watching that video, and I wished I could give that child nice clothes, shoes, and a wheelchair so he doesn't have to use his tummy to move around.

Mom, please send a wheelchair and nice clothes to that child in the video.

I love children so much, and I wish they could get good stuff like us.

Thank you, Mom, for loving these children who need your help, and thank you, God, for helping my mom achieve her goals in supporting these children with special needs."

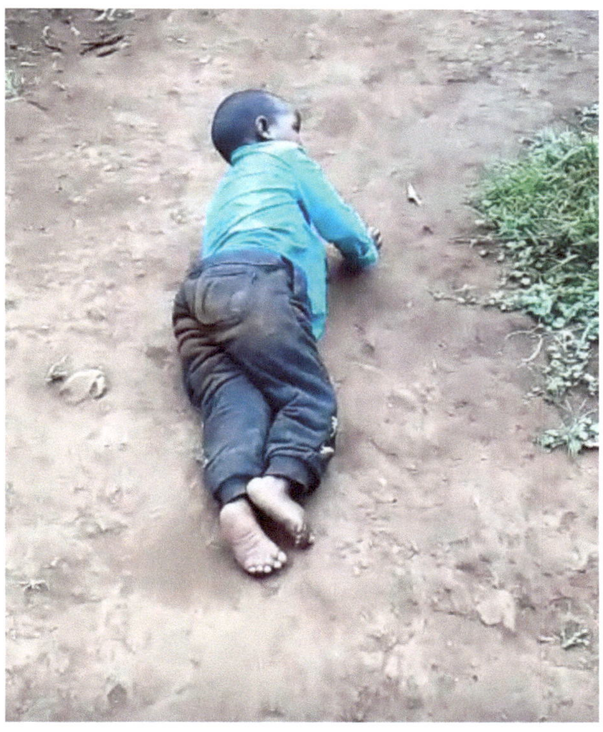

A picture of the child who made my sone Prince cry

SPECIAL MESSAGES FROM MOTHERS

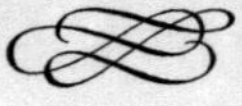

A Mother's Plea for Her Child

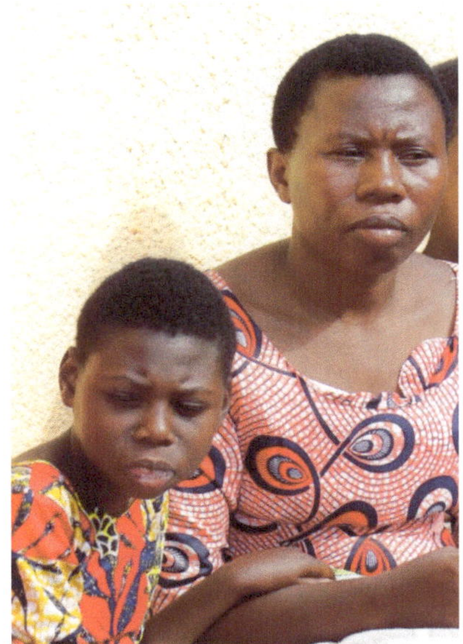

Sarafina

"My name is Sarafina and my daughter's name is Uwase Melissa.

My life turned upside down when I had my child with special needs. Since then, I have faced constant hurtful words from people in my village who call my child every sort of name. When other children see my child, they run away in fear. Some of my fellow women have even told me that I should starve my child until she dies, so I can move on with my life. But I did not listen to them because she is my gift from God.

I have suffered a great deal, but I will never give up on my child. I am calling on the government to hear our pain and provide the support we desperately need. We need access to the right medication, special diets, schools, diapers, pads, and any other resources that can help us care for our children.

A Mother's Struggle: Protecting My Daughter from the World's Cruelty.

My daughter is now 14 years old, but she still cries often and cannot feed herself, I am the only person who can be able to feed her and attend her care, she is just mine and sometimes I ask myself if anything ever happens to me, how can my daughter survive. Every day is a challenge, not only because of her needs but also because of the hurtful words I endure from those around me. There's one neighbor in particular who constantly says cruel things to me. She had a child with special needs too, but her child didn't survive. She blames me for my daughter's condition, saying it's my fault that her own child was born with special needs.

The pain of these words is unbearable at times. To protect my daughter from hearing such cruel things, I sometimes lock her inside the house. It breaks my heart to do this, but I want to shield her from the harshness of the world outside.

In moments like these, I remind myself that my daughter is my gift. She may face challenges that others do not understand, but she is a precious gift from God, and I will continue to love and protect her no matter what.

A Heartfelt Thank You to the International Community Center.

I want to thank the International Community Center (ICC) for coming to my rescue. The moment I joined other women in the group, I felt alive again. The group reminded me that I am not alone, and my child is not alone. ICC has done what no one else has—making us feel truly loved and cared for.

I can witness the goodness and generosity of the International Community Center. May God bless them abundantly for the incredible work they are doing. I have hope because I know there are still good people out there who can simply love you for who you are. My daughter, my family, and I are so grateful.

To anyone who can help, please remember our children. They deserve to be loved, cared for, and given the chance to live with dignity."

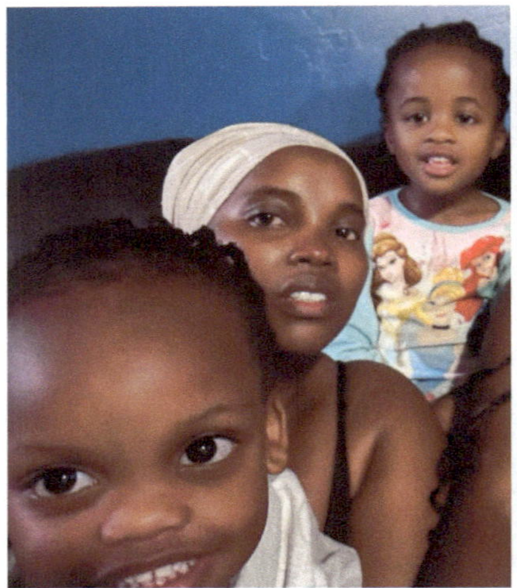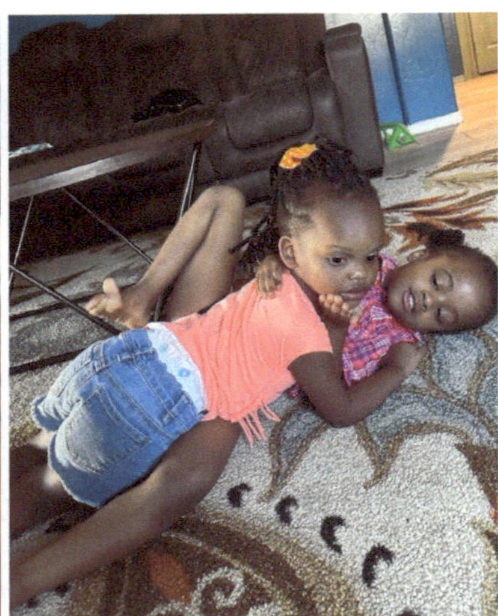

Jacqueline B. Hope

"First of all, I greet everyone who will read my story. My name is Jacqueline B. Hope. I am a Rwandan woman who lives in Arizona USA who has faced difficult life experiences. Since I was 6 years old, I found myself all alone with no mom, dad or siblings but God was by my side. I sympathize with anyone who has gone through painful experiences, which I will talk about here.

There is a Rwandan proverb that says, "Where you hang something, it will not fall." I am among those for whom it did not fall. I gave birth like others, and I have 4 children, but two of them were born with special needs known as Autism. It was not easy because they are the only family I have, both in front and behind me. But I live with it. It is not easy to live a life that is not stable.

And there's something I want to add here about Autism, it's hard to tell from the look that a child has Autism but deep inside we as parents know what our children go through on a daily basis, being judged at school, being judged in the stores and in public.

People calling you names that you don't know how to raise children with good manners and not knowing that the child they are judging has special needs now imagine having two children, siblings with Autism. Please pray for me. It's not easy for me and

honestly , I live like a crazy person because I am always running, taking them to places where they are taught how to speak for speech therapy, doctors appointments.

A child with this condition requires 100% assistance; they cannot help themselves at all, which is very difficult.

I want to take this opportunity to thank the U.S. government because we receive the support we need, although as parents, we always seek more help.

We are always trying to find additional help to see if they can get something out of life when we are no longer here.

Even though it's not easy, we combine it with prayer in this journey I've faced, along with a deep wound caused by the father of my children. He beat me and even told me that I was worthless, except for giving birth to "fools." These words stuck with me, and I lost sleep permanently. I am always running around looking for ways to help them. He finally left me because I had two children with special needs.

This story aims to encourage everyone who is hopeless and doesn't see how tomorrow will turn out. Be strong; the Lord knows you, especially parents in Africa who don't have anything to give to their children. You don't have even a diaper and have to leave your children alone at home to go find something to feed them. It is not easy, but take heart. Don't lose hope; the Lord knows you. We have also committed ourselves to be there for you as much as we can. Be strong; you are not alone.

In conclusion, I thank the U.S. government for the way it cares for people with special needs and gives them value, something some parents deny their own children.

I also ask other governments or any other country that doesn't care for people with special needs to take action because they are people like anyone else. If they receive help, at least the pain of the parents will decrease, and they will also be able to care for their other children, giving them the time they deserve. Because often, the whole heart is devoted to those with special needs, and the others end up feeling like orphans.

Finally, I ask that we join together to help stop the marginalization of people with special needs.

Thank you."

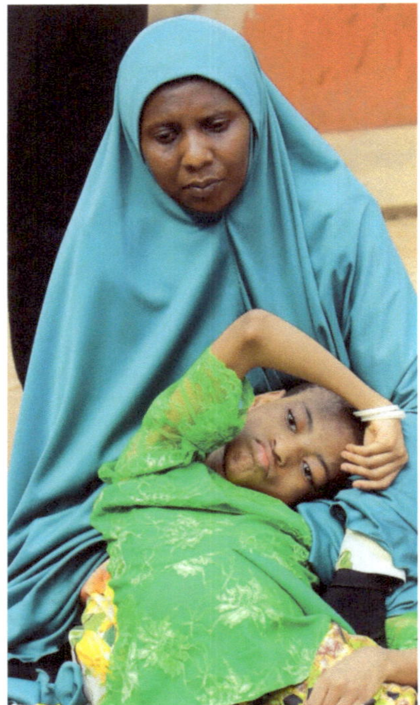

Esperance.

"My name is Esperance. I am a mother of a child with special needs; my daughter is 14 years old, and my journey has been filled with pain and heartbreak. When my husband found out that our child had special needs, he left us. His family turned against me, blaming me for our child's condition. My child has cerebral palsy; she can't sit, she can't move, and she can't stand.

The shame and judgment from others became so overwhelming that I began hiding my child, isolating us from neighbors and the people around us.

I have worked so hard all my life to provide for my family, but everything changed 14 years ago when my child was born. I went from being a provider to becoming a beggar, struggling every day to afford the medications, diapers, and food my child needs to survive.

I am crying out for help—not just for myself, but for all the mothers like me who are battling in silence. We need our governments to recognize our struggles and provide the support we so desperately need. We should not have to beg to give our children the care they deserve. We need financial assistance, healthcare, and resources so that we can focus on loving and supporting our children, rather than constantly worrying about how we will make it through another day.

After enduring so much pain in my life, I found Diana, the founder of ICC. She listened to me and advised me to gather other mothers like me, who have children with special needs, so we could create a group where we can meet with our children and support one another. I did what she told me, and now we are a group of many women, and I am the team leader. Others want to join us because our support group is doing an incredible job, and ICC is making a tremendous impact on our lives. Our lives have changed because of the International Community Center, and we are forever grateful. We are now thinking of reaching out to those who are very abandoned in rural areas so we can keep spreading the word until our government recognizes us. We will not stop until we reach other children with special needs. Let's be the voice so we can be heard by our leaders. Our children need us, and we need your support to make it happen. As the leader of this women's group, I am speaking on behalf of every woman in this group.

A Collective Call for Support

I am speaking on behalf of my fellow women in this group, mothers of special needs children. We ask you to listen to us and understand the heavy burdens we carry every day. We love our children deeply, but the challenges we face are overwhelming. We need your help to ease some of these burdens so we can focus on what matters mostâ€"caring for our children.

Please hear our plea and take action to support us. By providing the necessary resources and assistance, you allow us to give our children the care and love they deserve. Together, we can make a difference in their lives.

To all those who can hear my plea, please help us. We are mothers who are fighting for our childrenâ€™s lives, but we cannot do it alone."

A Message from a Parent

A Parent's Journey: From Struggle to Hope

Here's a heartfelt message from a parent with a child with special needs in the USA. However, this parent had her child in Africa, and she knows what her fellow women go through. She wants to encourage them not to give up. Their children are blessings, and she wishes for them to stay strong. Maybe one day, their lives and their children's lives may change as hers did. She no longer has to worry about hospital bills, feeding her child, or diapers anymore.

"As a parent of a child with special needs in Africa, my journey has been incredibly difficult. For years, I traveled from one country to another in search of treatment for my child, facing countless challenges along the way. In Africa, there was no government support, no accessible healthcare, and no resources to help me care for my child. I felt completely alone, burdened with the heavy weight of trying to provide for my child's needs without the necessary support.

But everything changed when I came to the United States of America. Here, my child finally received the support, healthcare, and resources that were so desperately needed. The love, respect, and support that the U.S. government shows to parents and children with special needs have been a lifeline for us. I am deeply grateful for the compassion and care we have found here.

To the leaders of African nations, I implore you to raise awareness for children with special needs and to provide financial support to their parents. These children deserve to be treated with dignity and respect, and their parents should not have to choose between their child's health and their own survival. With proper support, parents can dedicate their time and energy to caring for their children without the constant worry about affording medications, diapers, and special diets.

It is time for African leaders to step up and ensure that all children, regardless of their abilities, have access to the care and support they need to thrive.

Dear Fellow Women,

I was in your shoes some years back, facing the same struggles and challenges. I want to encourage you to stay strong and fight for your children until you win. I came to the United States of America because of my child with special needs, and I had other children who were not special needs. That child is your gift—you never know the places you will go because of your gift. Love them, cherish them, and don't give up on them.

I love you all."

A MESSAGE TO OUR READERS: HOW YOU CAN MAKE A DIFFERENCE

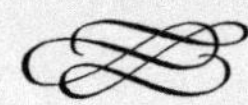

Dear Readers,

Thank you for taking the time to read *I Am Your Gift*. Your support means the world to us, and we hope that the stories and experiences shared within these pages have touched your heart as deeply as they have touched ours.

As you may have noticed, throughout this book, we have included the names and photos of some of the incredible children who are part of our program. Each of these children has a unique story, full of both challenges and potential. They are the true inspiration behind this book, and they are also in need of your support.

If you feel moved to make a difference in the life of a child, we invite you to consider becoming a sponsor. Sponsorship allows you to directly support the needs of a child—whether it's providing them with education, healthcare, or the special resources they require to thrive. Your sponsorship can help ensure that these children receive the care and opportunities they deserve.

How to Sponsor a Child:

1. **Review the Children's Profiles:** As you read through the book, take note of the children's names and stories that resonate with you. Their profiles include their needs and how your support can help.
2. **Contact Us:** Reach out to us using the contact information provided at the end of this book or visit our website. We will guide you through the sponsorship process and provide you with more detailed information on how your contributions will be used.
3. **Build a Connection:** As a sponsor, you will have the opportunity to stay connected with the child you support. You can receive updates, letters, and even photos, seeing firsthand the impact of your generosity.
4. **Make a Lasting Impact:** Sponsorship is not just about providing financial support—it's about giving a child hope and the chance to build a brighter future. Your kindness can transform lives, offering these children the love and care they need to grow and succeed.

Thank you for considering this meaningful way to give back. Together, we can create a world where every child, regardless of their circumstances, has the opportunity to realize their full potential.

With heartfelt gratitude,

Diana Uwera

Some pictures of our beautiful children

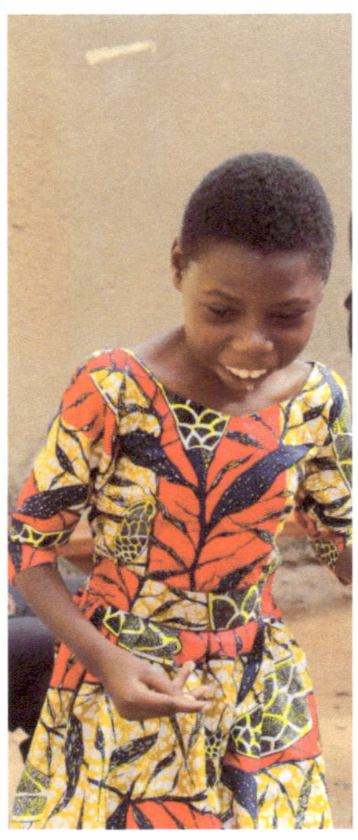

Uwase Melissa. Non verbal and cerebral palsyÂ

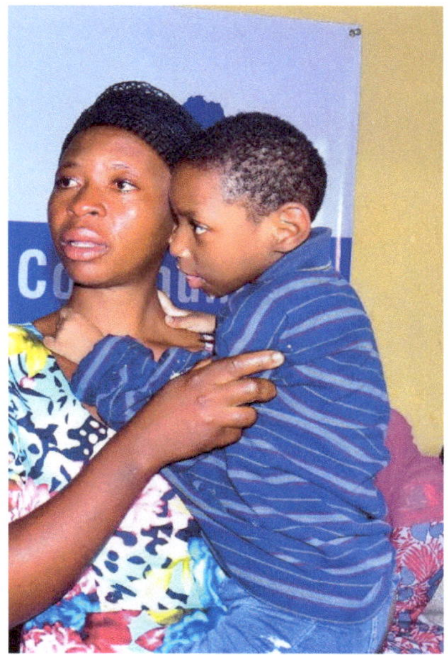

Gabiro Antique- Deceased mother. Non verbalÂ Cerebral palsyÂ

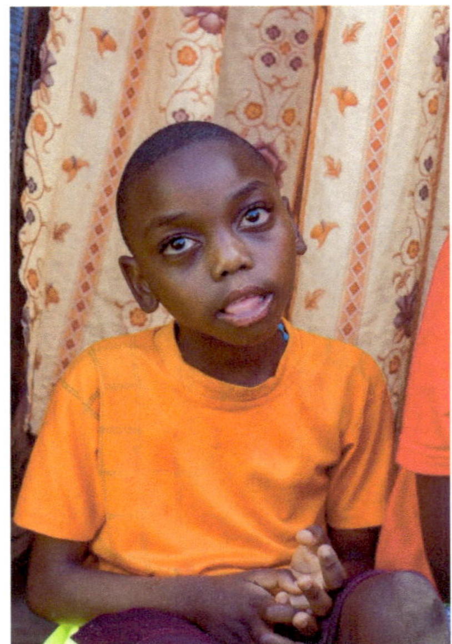

Irakoze Armeri Non verbal and cerebral palsy.

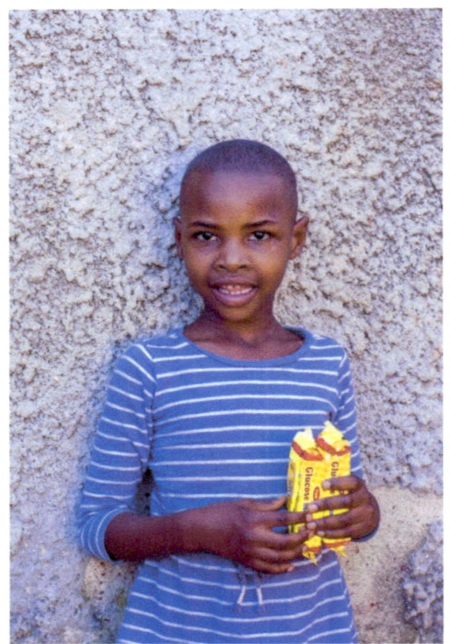

Agasaro Uwase Amila. Non verbal and Autism.

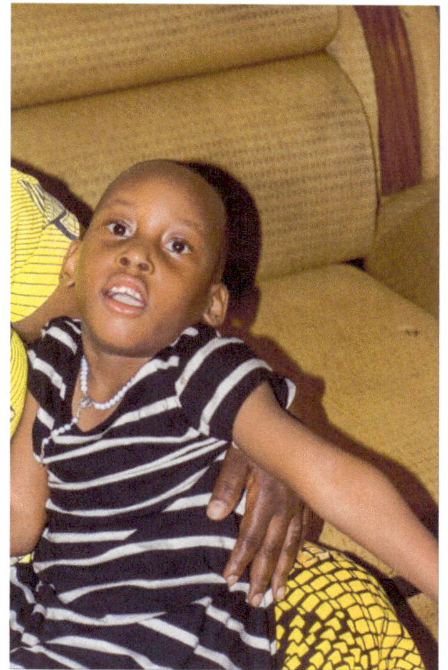

Umutesi Jessica. Non verbal and cerebral palsy.

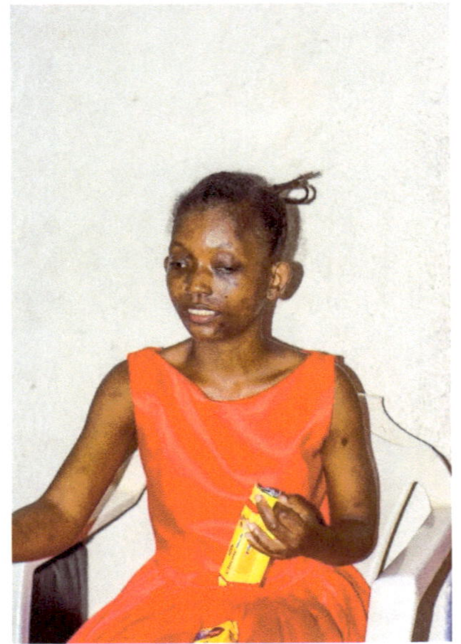

Mutoni Shemusa. Down SyndromeÂ

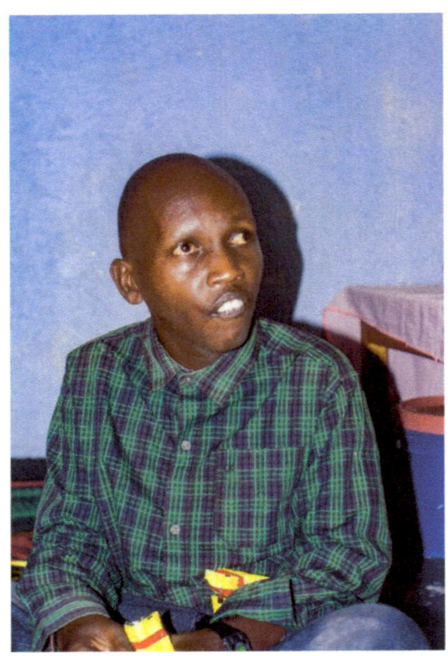

Mbarushimana Hamuza. Down Syndrome.

A CALL TO ACTION

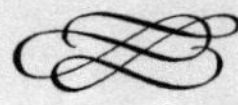

As you reach the final pages of "I Am Your Gift," I want to leave you with a message of hope, purpose, and a call to action. Throughout this journey, we've explored the challenges, joys, and immense value of children with special needs. We've celebrated their unique gifts and the profound impact they have on our lives. Now, as we look to the future, it's time to think about what more we can do together to support these incredible children.

As you turn these last pages, you'll see the faces of some of the children who are part of our program. Each smile, each expression, tells a story of resilience, courage, and the potential waiting to be unlocked with the right support. These children are the reason this book exists— they are the heartbeat of this mission.

But there is so much more to be done. Many of these children, and others like them, face daily struggles that no child should have to endure. They need access to education, healthcare, and therapies that can help them thrive. They need safe environments where they can grow and learn, and they need the love and support of people who believe in them.

This is where you come in.

To the donors, sponsors, and all the good-hearted people out there reading this: I invite you to join us in this cause. Your support can make a world of difference in the lives of these children. Whether it's through a donation, sponsorship, or simply spreading the word about our mission, your contribution is invaluable.

Together, we can create a brighter future for these children. A future where they are not only seen and heard but where they are given every opportunity to reach their full potential. By standing with us, you are becoming part of a movement that champions the rights, dignity, and worth of every child with special needs.

Let us unite in love and action, so that each of these children can shine as brightly as they were meant to. Thank you for being part of this journey and for considering how you can help. Your kindness and generosity will leave a lasting impact on these children's lives and on the world we all share.

With deepest gratitude and hope,

Diana Uwera